INTERMITTENT FASTING FOR WOMEN OVER 50 MADE EASY

A BEGINNER'S GUIDE TO SAFELY MAINTAIN A HEALTHY WEIGHT, HORMONAL BALANCE, INCREASE ENERGY LEVELS, AND MENTAL CLARITY WHILE AVOIDING COMMON PITFALLS

GRACE ERICKSON

CONTENTS

Introduction   5

1. THE ABCS OF INTERMITTENT FASTING   11
   Intermittent Fasting: The Basics   12
   Common Misconceptions About Intermittent
   Fasting   19
   Common Intermittent Fasting Mistakes   24

2. AGE GRACEFULLY WITH INTERMITTENT
   FASTING   29
   The Golden Years: Metabolism and Hormonal Shifts   30
   The Science Behind Intermittent Fasting   36
   Achieving Hormonal Harmony Through
   Intermittent Fasting   39
   Cognitive Benefits of Intermittent Fasting   41

3. GETTING STARTED WITH INTERMITTENT
   FASTING   43
   Suitable Intermittent Fasting Methods for Women
   Over 50   44
   Fasting Styles   49
   Guidelines for Safely Starting Intermittent Fasting   52

4. POWERING UP YOUR ENERGY LEVELS AND
   MENTAL CLARITY   61
   The Psychological Relationship Between
   Intermittent Fasting, Energy Levels, and Mental
   Clarity   62
   Intermittent Fasting and Metabolism, Brain
   Function, and Overall Cognitive Performance   63
   Research and Relevant Studies Supporting the
   Connection Between Intermittent Fasting, Energy
   Levels, and Mental Clarity   66
   Understanding the Relevance of the Research
   Findings on Intermittent Fasting   68
   Strategies for Using Intermittent Fasting to Enhance
   Mental Focus   69

Dealing With Fatigue and Brain Fog   73
Practical Tips to Overcome Challenges   75

5. THE WEIGH TO WELLNESS   79
   Intermittent Fasting and Weight Management   80
   Research that Supports Intermittent Fasting's Role in
   Weight Management   82
   Strategies for Weight Maintenance Through
   Intermittent Fasting   83
   Exercise Suggestions for Women Over 50   85
   Tips for Starting an Exercise Routine   93

6. NOURISHING YOUR FASTING BODY   97
   The Importance of Nutrition in Intermittent Fasting   98
   Listening to Your Body's Needs   101
   What to Eat During Eating Windows for Optimal
   Health   107

7. HEART-HEALTHY RECIPES FOR INTERMITTENT
   FASTING   111
   Nourishing and Delicious Savory Recipes   112
   Ingredients and Benefits   147
   Tips for Choosing Ingredients   149

8. YOUR 28-DAY PATH TO SUCCESS   151
   The 28-Day Meal Planning Made Simple   151
   Fasting Forward: Adjusting for Success   155

   Conclusion   159
   References   163

INTRODUCTION

For me, reaching 50 wasn't just a milestone. It was also a stark realization that my body had been giving warning signals that I hadn't been listening to. It was a cancer diagnosis that immediately stopped all the complacency and forced me to confront my health head-on. My fears of the disease were fought by a fierce desire to live, which led me to discover intermittent fasting. This dietary pattern helped me overcome the physical and emotional whirl-wind of cancer treatment. Intermittent fasting didn't offer me an instant solution, but my recovery gradually became a reality as my body got used to the practice. This book shares with you the science behind intermittent fasting and the numerous benefits that you can derive from engaging in the practice, backed by scientific findings. I have specifically tailor-made different fasting approaches to meet your unique needs as a woman over 50.

We'll explore the hormone fluctuations and metabolism shifts that you are experiencing, and the specific benefits that intermittent fasting offers during this important life stage. It's true that while both men and women experience increased vulnerability to disease with aging, research suggests that women may face a higher risk for certain chronic conditions (Fiacco et al., 2020). This phenomenon can be attributed to several factors, including hormones, genetics, and immune system differences.

Do you stare in the mirror and see disturbing lines where youthful contours once were? Does the societal spotlight that you used to glow in now seem dim and focused on younger faces and figures? Are you constantly anxious about remembering details because of memory fog or worried about aches and pains that have become unwelcome companions? My dear friend, I feel your pain, and I am here to assure you that you are not alone. Trust me, I know all too well the struggles of trying to find your way through a world seemingly obsessed with youth while you gracefully age.

INTRODUCING THE GRACE FRAMEWORK!

In this book, you'll discover a wealth of strategies that are designed to empower you on your journey toward vibrant health, particularly as you age. Let's take a peek at the valuable insights and tools waiting to be explored. These are presented to you using the GRACE framework, which is decoded as follows:

- **G (Groundwork):** I begin by building a solid foundation for the book. This stage is covered in Chapter 1 and breaks down the essentials of what intermittent fasting is all about. We'll explore the potential benefits that the practice offers while debunking some common myths to ultimately equip you with the knowledge that you need to walk the fasting journey with clarity and confidence.

- **R (Revitalize)**: This part is covered in Chapter 2, and the section addresses how your metabolism might slow down, and your hormonal balance might be disturbed as you age. I will explain how these shifts impact your weight and overall well-being. We'll also explore how intermittent fasting can help you achieve a healthier hormonal balance, thus managing your weight effectively.
- **A (Adapt)**: In this section, I'll walk you through different intermittent fasting methods and help you discover the one that aligns best with your lifestyle and goals. It's not just about choosing a method; it's also about preparing your mind and body for the journey. Chapter 3 covers all this.
- **C (Cultivate)**: Chapters 4 and 5 are about exploring strategies to keep your energy levels soaring and your mind sharp throughout the day. We also talk about weight management and physical exercises, both practically and sustainably.
- **E (Enrich)**: In the final section stretching through Chapters 6, 7, and 8, you'll discover how to eat mindfully, choose heart-healthy food options, and make intermittent fasting work with your unique dietary needs. I've also included a handy 28-day meal planner to help you along.

PROOF THAT INTERMITTENT FASTING REALLY DOES WORK!

The success of intermittent fasting is practically proven. Instead of just relying on generic statements about the practice, let me share with you just a few of the many real-life stories of women who transformed their lives through intermittent fasting:

- **Roxanne's testimony**: Roxanne, always lean and active, found herself unknowingly gaining weight over the years. Despite her efforts to trim down her body frame, the scale wouldn't reflect any changes in her weight. Frustrated, she began exploring various options and discovered intermittent fasting through her friends. Intrigued by the practice, she adopted a simple 16/8 approach, eating only between 11 a.m. and 7 p.m. Using this approach combined with a balanced diet, she shed 10 pounds in just a couple of months. Her story, like many others, demonstrates the potential of intermittent fasting to achieve healthy goals (Harlan, 2016).

- **Jeethah's story**: Jeethah's frequent dizziness and falls because of a lack of balance were a constant reminder of her out-of-control blood sugar levels. She'd tried medication and strict diets, but none of these seemed to work. When Jeethah heard about intermittent fasting, she wasted no time in adopting the practice. In just a few weeks, the mental fog began clearing away from her mind. Dizziness became a thing of the past, and her body was filled with renewed energy. When she went for her medical review, the doctor confirmed what Jeethah already knew: her diabetes was gone for good (Stevens, 2019).

- **Sandy's testimony**: Sandy's grip had been crippled by rheumatoid arthritis, which made her struggle even with simple tasks. She felt a glimmer of hope when a friend suggested intermittent fasting to her. Embracing the 5:2 approach, she fasted twice a week, enjoying her meals only within limited windows. Two months went by, and then suddenly, her fingers, which were once stiff and swollen, began moving with greater ease (Quora, 2019).

GET TO KNOW THE AUTHOR

Having received a stage 4 breast cancer diagnosis and overcome the condition, the author, Grace Erickson, is happy to share with you how she beat the effects of chemotherapy through intermittent fasting, healthy dietary consumption, and exercise. Come along and join the 57-year-old victor on this empowering journey, and let's reclaim your youthful vibrancy through intermittent fasting! Let's begin.

THE ABCS OF INTERMITTENT FASTING

A re you tired of diets that leave you feeling deprived and frustrated? Or better yet, do you want to unlock a secret weapon for weight management, boosted energy, and a sharper mind? Are you stressed, sleep-deprived, and wondering if your "normal" self will ever come back to you after 50? Well, worry no longer; I hear you. What if I told you that there was a simple approach that could help you manage stress, sleep soundly, and rediscover your youthful zest for life? Forget all the restrictive diets and quick fixes that leave you unsatisfied, and discover the world of intermittent fasting that is tailored particularly for amazing women over 50 like you!

This chapter enlightens you on some intermittent fasting considerations that are specifically designed for the unique needs of mature women like you. It also addresses intermittent fasting's essential elements that you need to consider before starting the routine, including its benefits, misconceptions, and the common mistakes that you need to avoid. These factors represent the "**Groundwork**" section of the "**GRACE**" framework covered in this book, which is represented by the letter "**G**" in the acronym. If you are ready to reclaim your good health and feel your best, then this chapter unveils a powerful tool that can help you achieve your goals without restrictive diets or endless hours at the gym. Wave goodbye to fatigue, and let's welcome a revitalized and empowered you. The useful nuggets that I share in this chapter will help you to feel good, look great, and age gracefully and sustainably. Let's explore further.

INTERMITTENT FASTING: THE BASICS

The dietary approach of intermittent fasting avoids the extremeness of calorie counting and restrictive meal plans. It isn't a "diet" in the traditional sense, but rather a unique approach to shifting your eating schedule instead of focusing on the food that you eat. It is more focused on the benefits that your body gets from giving your digestive system a well-deserved rest. By alternating between your eating and fasting intervals, you enhance your metabolic system's ability to support your general well-being and health. Now, you may be wondering, but how does intermittent fasting actually work? Well, you choose a fasting schedule that suits you and then be sure to stick to it. Some popular fasting methods involve limiting your eating window to just a few hours within a 24-hour period. Alternatively, you may engage in a 5:2 approach, where you eat normally for five days and then restrict your calories on two non-consecutive days. The idea behind this strategy is to emphasize when you eat instead of focusing on what you consume. Intermittent fasting is all about giving your body enough time to process food efficiently and then reaping the benefits of gentle detoxification during the fasting periods.

The Main Benefits of Intermittent Fasting

Intermittent fasting adds many health benefits to your body. In this section, I go with you into the healthy transformation that happens within your body when you embrace this dietary approach. Remember, these are just some of the many potential merits of engaging in the practice, more of which you will realize from your personal experiences once you start your routine. Also, before embarking on this dietary practice, professional medical consultations will be crucial for ensuring that it aligns with your individual needs and health conditions. Let's flow together as I highlight some of intermittent fasting's merits, including:

Weight Loss

Counting your calories regularly can become extremely tedious. Intermittent fasting, thereby, comes with a different solution. Restricting the period when you may eat results in less calorie intake. This aids in healthy weight loss. Intermittent fasting's weight-loss benefits have been backed by numerous studies. A 2020 review that analyzed 25 controlled trials found that an average weight loss of between three and eight percent resulted from various fasting methods over a period ranging from two months to a year. Some individuals were even reported to have experienced greater body mass reductions than what these figures show (Gunnars, 2021).

Compared to calorie-restricted diets, intermittent fasting results in similar weight loss but without requiring strict calorie counting. Moreover, it appears to be particularly effective in reducing abdominal fat, which is a significant risk factor for the onset of chronic diseases. While the exploration of the exact mechanisms that are involved is still being conducted, researchers believe that intermittent fasting promotes weight loss by decreasing calorie intake, boosting metabolism, and regulating hunger hormones (Gunnars, 2021).

Reduced Insulin Resistance

Insulin resistance, which is a key player in many chronic diseases, can be tackled with intermittent fasting. By giving your body breaks from processing food, you improve insulin sensitivity, leading to better blood sugar regulation. Studies reveal promising results in support of intermittent fasting's ability to help prevent the onset of chronic diseases. In 2019, research showed significant improvements in insulin sensitivity across various dietary approaches, with reductions in insulin levels during intermittent fasting of up to 25% (Gunnars, 2021). Notably, these improvements were independent of weight loss, thereby suggesting that the benefits of intermittent fasting directly impact insulin regulation. Research also points to increased insulin receptor activity and reduced inflammation as potential mechanisms behind this effect (Gunnars, 2021). As this existing evidence suggests, mitigating the risks that are associated with conditions like type 2 diabetes and improving insulin sensitivity are merits that can be brought about by practicing intermittent fasting consistently.

Decreased Inflammation

Chronic inflammation intensifies various health issues in women over 50. Intermittent fasting helps to fight this by reducing inflammation markers throughout your body. This effect lowers your risk of developing conditions like heart disease and arthritis. With the power of controlled fasting, your body can start feeling lighter, both physically and mentally. It has been found that various fasting methods led to significant reductions in key inflammatory markers like C-reactive protein and interleukin-6. Additionally, a study also observed that alternate-day fasting specifically decreased gut inflammation, and the practice likely offers benefits for inflammatory bowel diseases (Johns Hopkins Medicine, 2021). These benefits are attributed to reduced oxidative stress, improved gut microbiome composition, and the activation of cellular repair pathways. Gut microbiomes are the viruses, bacteria, and fungi that inhabit your digestive tract and assist in the breakdown of food. With research still ongoing, these findings still suggest that incorporating intermittent fasting into your lifestyle can be a strategic move to combat inflammation and lower your risk of developing chronic diseases.

Reducing Levels of Bad Cholesterol

High cholesterol acts as a silent health threat to women over 50. Significantly reduced levels of "bad" low-density lipoprotein (LDL) and enhanced production of "good" high-density lipoprotein (HDL) cholesterol can both be achieved through practicing intermittent fasting. This double action creates a healthier lipid profile that protects your heart and circulatory system. Research has found that various fasting methods led to significant reductions in LDL cholesterol, with some individuals experiencing decreases of up to 25%. Interestingly, even short-term fasting cycles were also shown to be effective. A 2017 study observed a decrease in LDL after just eight weeks of alternate-day fasting (Fiacco et al., 2020). It is believed that these impacts are due to the increased breakdown and excretion, along with decreased production, of "bad cholesterol" by the liver. Additionally, fasting appears to benefit "good" HDL cholesterol by creating a more favorable lipid profile overall.

Decreased Risk Factors for Heart Disease

The benefits for your heart won't stop at cholesterol. Intermittent fasting reduces blood pressure, improves blood vessel function, and decreases inflammation, thereby creating a powerful shield against heart disease. Heart disease is the leading cause of death globally. The research findings on intermittent fasting offer positive indications. It has been found that various fasting methods led to improvements in multiple heart disease risk factors, including reductions in blood pressure, blood sugar levels, and triglycerides (Gunnars, 2021). These factors are the major causes of heart disease. Additionally, observations that alternate-day fasting specifically improved blood vessel function, which is a key factor in preventing heart attacks, have also been made. These results have shown that improved insulin sensitivity, reduced inflammation, and favorable changes in cholesterol levels contribute to reduced risk factors for developing heart disease.

Improved Brain Health

Intermittent fasting nourishes your brain, thereby promoting the growth of new cells and enhancing memory function. This mindful eating pattern allows you to experience improved focus, sharper thinking, and a revitalized mind. Research analysis on animal models has discovered that various fasting methods increase the production of brain-derived neurotrophic factor (BDNF). BDNF is a protein that is crucial for nerve cell growth and survival, which improves cognitive function and memory (Johns Hopkins Medicine, 2021). Improved learning and memory performance were also observed in people who practiced alternate-day fasting for three months. These effects stem from increased brain cell repair, reduced inflammation, and improved blood flow to the brain that occurs during intermittent fasting, thus reducing the risk of developing neurodegenerative diseases.

It Promotes Anti-Aging Effects

While aging is inevitable, its effects can be mitigated. Intermittent fasting has shown potential anti-aging properties by promoting cellular repair. This dietary approach allows you to relive your youthful nature by feeling vibrant and energetic. While the fountain of youth might remain elusive, research suggests that various fasting methods extend the lifespan and improve the health span of different organisms. These fasting approaches achieve this by activating cellular repair mechanisms and reducing oxidative stress. A research study conducted in 2019 observed that alternate-day fasting improved DNA repair in human cells, which is a critical component in preventing age-related cellular damage (Johns Hopkins Medicine, 2021). While human trials are still being carried out, the current validation of findings confirms that incorporating intermittent fasting into your lifestyle could help slow down cellular aging, thereby improving your resistance to age-related diseases and contributing to a healthier and longer life.

Intermittent Fasting Versus Other Methods

While all dietary approaches essentially aim for improved health, intermittent fasting stands apart from other methods in its unique methodology and health benefits. Let's review some of intermittent fasting's key differences:

- **Calorie counting:** This method carefully tracks your intake to achieve a specific calorie deficit for weight loss. While effective for some people, it can be restrictive, and tedious, and may create an unhealthy obsession with numbers. Intermittent fasting, on the other hand, focuses on the times that you eat, not just the amount of food, thereby offering more flexibility and improving metabolism through strategic fasting periods.
- **3-day diet:** This restrictive diet promises rapid weight loss in just three days by severely limiting calorie intake. While it might lead to quick weight loss, this approach is unsustainable, nutrient-deficient, and can backfire by causing rebound weight gain and other potential health

risks (Shah, 2022). In contrast, intermittent fasting promotes long-term healthy habits and avoids extreme calorie restriction, thereby allowing a sustainable and balanced approach to weight management.

- **Body reset diet:** This trendy program often involves eliminating entire food groups or following specific purification techniques to detoxify the body. While the concept of removing toxins from your body is appealing, there is little scientific evidence to support these claims. As such, restrictive diets can be unhealthy, as they may withhold vital nutrients from your body. Intermittent fasting, on the other hand, focuses on nourishing your body with healthy foods within designated eating windows. This naturally prompts cellular repair and detoxification processes.

- **Mediterranean diet:** This heart-healthy eating pattern emphasizes fruits, vegetables, whole grains, and healthy fats, thereby offering numerous health benefits beyond weight management. While similar to its focus on wholesome foods, intermittent fasting complements this approach by adding the element of timed eating. This enhances the benefits of a Mediterranean diet by experiencing its metabolic effects.

- **Detox diet:** Similar to body reset diets, this approach often involves restrictive eating or body cleansing routines with unverified detoxification claims. Intermittent fasting, however, doesn't support these unsubstantiated assertions. The natural fasting periods inherent to intermittent fasting help to support your body's own detoxification processes without resorting to extreme measures like nutrient deprivation.

COMMON MISCONCEPTIONS ABOUT INTERMITTENT FASTING

Intermittent fasting has gained traction over the last few years, but misconceptions continuously cloud its full potential. Let's clear the air on some of these myths:

Myth 1

Your metabolism is slowed down by fasting.

Reality

Studies suggest the opposite. Short-term fasting is actually thought to boost your metabolism, thereby helping you burn more calories during your periods of inactivity (Nazish, 2024).

Myth 2

Fasting makes you lose muscle.

Reality

Muscle loss primarily occurs from inactivity, not controlled fasting. Prioritizing protein intake and incorporating strength training during eating windows helps preserve muscle mass.

Myth 3

Fasting causes nutrient deficiencies.

Reality

With careful planning and mindful food choices during eating windows, you can ensure that you meet your nutritional needs.

Consulting a registered dietitian can help you personalize your fasting approach.

Myth 4

Fasting is unsafe.

Reality

For most healthy individuals, properly implementing intermittent fasting is safe. However, it is crucial to engage in professional medical consultations before starting the practice, particularly if you have suffered from any pre-existing health conditions before.

Myth 5

Fasting is only about weight loss.

Reality

Beyond weight management, intermittent fasting offers various benefits for heart health, brain function, inflammation reduction, and many other body improvements.

Myth 6

Fasting harms your brain, mental alertness, and focus.

Reality

Studies suggest that you will experience improved cognitive function, mental clarity, and focus during fasting periods (Nazish, 2024).

Myth 7

There's no scientific evidence for fasting's effectiveness.

Reality

Numerous studies support the benefits of intermittent fasting for various health markers. While research is still ongoing, the available scientific claims are encouraging (Nazish, 2024).

Myth 8

Intermittent fasting means skipping breakfast.

Reality

Intermittent fasting is just about when you eat and not necessarily about skipping meals. Choose an eating window that fits your lifestyle, regardless of whether or not it includes breakfast.

Myth 9

Fasting is a miracle cure for weight loss.

Reality

Intermittent fasting is an effective aid for body improvement. However, it does not work magically. Weight loss depends on your overall dietary choices, exercise, and other individual lifestyle factors.

Myth 10

All intermittent fasting is the same.

Reality

Different intermittent fasting methods exist, like the 16:8 and 5:2 approaches. Choose the one that aligns with your preferences, or consult a medical professional for guidance.

Myth 11

Fasting is good for everyone.

Reality

Intermittent fasting might not be suitable for everyone, especially pregnant or breastfeeding women, individuals with certain health conditions, or those with disordered eating histories. You need to obtain expert medical counsel before starting the practice if you have experienced any of the aforementioned issues before.

Myth 12

You can eat anything during the eating window.

Reality

During your eating window, you are advised to focus on nutrient-dense and whole, unprocessed foods to optimize your health and well-being. Intermittent fasting's benefits can be negated by eating processed foods and excessive calorie intake within your designated feeding windows.

Myth 13

Water intake is restricted during fasting windows.

Reality

Staying hydrated during intermittent fasting is crucial. You should drink plenty of water and unsweetened tea, or black coffee, during fasting periods.

Myth 14

Fasting puts your body into starvation mode.

Reality

This is a common misconception that prevents many people from adopting or beginning the practice altogether. Your body adapts to fasting by utilizing stored energy sources efficiently, not by entering starvation mode.

Myth 15

Your brain needs a constant supply of dietary glucose.

Reality

While a constant supply of glucose helps to boost mental function, your brain can adapt to using ketones for energy during intermittent fasting. Ketones are molecules that are produced by your liver during periods of low carbohydrate or sugar intake that are particularly effective in enhancing cognitive function.

To be completely sure that you bust any intermittent fasting myths, get informed counsel before starting any new dietary approach, particularly if you have pre-existing health issues. You can, therefore, make informed decisions about whether or not to partake in intermittent fasting by separating the myths from the facts.

COMMON INTERMITTENT FASTING MISTAKES

We all stumble sometimes during important activities, and intermittent fasting is no exception. Whether you're just starting or you have been practicing this dietary approach for a while, remember that mistakes are part of the journey. Here are some of the common intermittent fasting mistakes that people usually make, and some friendly tips are listed beside each of them to help you steer clear of these common pitfalls:

- **Choosing the wrong program:** Not all fasting methods are created equal. Consider your lifestyle, preferences, and health goals before fasting. For personalized guidance, you may talk to a dietician or doctor prior to commencing the practice.
- **Overlooking your personal habits:** Don't force yourself to commit to an approach that doesn't suit your lifestyle. Choose a fasting schedule that fits your daily routine and commitments. Remember, flexibility is key to long-term intermittent fasting success.
- **You don't make a smooth transition:** Going all the way into intermittent fasting right from the beginning isn't for everyone. I advise you to start gradually, maybe just skipping dessert or delaying breakfast by an hour. Also, be sure to listen to your body and adjust the approach as needed.
- **Following an excessively strict diet:** Avoid rigid restrictions and extreme calorie deficits during intermittent fasting. During your eating windows,

remember to focus on nourishing your body with whole foods and unprocessed varieties.

- **Choosing unsuitable dietary options:** Remember to prioritize nutrient-dense options like lean proteins, healthy fats, vegetables, and fruits. Avoid junk foods that are normally a temptation during your feasting windows.
- **Consuming too many calories:** During your eating windows, taking mindful food portions is essential. The nutritional value of the food you take is what matters more than the portion sizes.
- **Drinking soda and beverages:** Avoid taking soda, juice, and sweetened drinks during your fast. During this period, drink plenty of water, black coffee, or unsweetened tea to stay hydrated and avoid blood sugar spikes.
- **Forgetting to hydrate and not keeping track of water intake:** Water is your best friend during intermittent fasting. Set reminders throughout the day to stay hydrated, especially during fasting periods. Track your water intake and aim for at least eight glasses daily.
- **Breaking your fast with too little nutrition:** Don't starve yourself during intermittent fasting. Take a balanced meal that is rich in protein, fiber, and healthy fats to satiate your hunger and energize your body when you finally break your fast.
- **Eating too much when you break your fast:** Remember, overeating, even healthy foods, can cancel out intermittent fasting's benefits. Pay attention to your body's hunger signals and stop eating when you are comfortably full.
- **Unknowingly breaking your fast:** Watch out for hidden sugars and additives that can unknowingly break your fast. Read food labels carefully, and stick to healthy food options.

- **Breaking a fast with low-protein, low-fiber foods:** When you break your fast, skip the refined carbs and sugary treats. Prioritize protein, fiber, and healthy fats for a balanced and satisfying meal to break your fast.
- **Going too extreme:** Sustainability is key during intermittent fasting. Don't push yourself too hard with overly aggressive fasting schedules or calorie restrictions. Start slow and gradually increase the intensity as you adapt to the practice.
- **Having caffeine withdrawals:** Wean yourself off caffeine intake gradually if you are a coffee lover. Stick to unsweetened coffee or tea during fasting windows to minimize withdrawal symptoms.
- **Being too rigid:** Don't be afraid to adjust your fasting plan as needed. Many life events and health conditions can happen to you that may require a shift in your fasting approach. Remain attentive to your body's needs, and be flexible enough to tweak your fasting approach whenever necessary.
- **Not exercising:** Regular physical activity boosts your metabolism and overall health, even during fasting periods. Aim for at least 30 minutes of physical exercise each day, and choose only the activities that you enjoy.
- **Engaging in an intense workout at the wrong time:** Your energy levels during intermittent fasting are worth noting. During your fasting window, opting for gentler activities like walking or yoga and then scheduling more intense workouts within your feeding period will be quite helpful.
- **Lack of sufficient sleep:** Prioritize getting quality sleep every night. To regulate your hormones and optimize organ recovery, aim for between seven and eight hours of sleep a night. This will support your fasting journey.

- **Giving up:** We all have setbacks, but don't let a stumble derail your progress. Get back on track and remember that progress, not perfection, is the ultimate goal of intermittent fasting.

This chapter has enlightened you on the basics of intermittent fasting, including how to conduct the practice and its immediate and long-term benefits. The benefits of intermittent fasting include improved mental clarity, a reduction in inflammation, and a lowered risk of developing chronic conditions like heart disease. The chapter also highlighted the comparative advantages of intermittent fasting against what is offered by other dietary methods, like calorie counting. Common myths about intermittent fasting were also busted by providing facts about the practice. These include the misconceptions that fasting is unsafe and that there is no scientific evidence to support the benefits of the practice. This chapter also highlighted the common pitfalls that are usually faced when practicing intermittent fasting while also giving remedies to overcome each pitfall. Once you understand these factors, it becomes more likely that you will enjoy intermittent fasting's full benefits, thereby enhancing your likelihood of aging gracefully. In the following chapter, let me walk you through the scientific facts and details behind these benefits.

AGE GRACEFULLY WITH INTERMITTENT FASTING

Fae Olson is one of the people who will bet on the effectiveness of intermittent fasting, especially after experiencing her own share of its advantages. Fae was introduced to intermittent fasting by her daughter, and she decided to give it a try in her early 70s (Olson, 2021). Not only did Fae lose weight from 141 to 114 pounds, but there were more "aha!" moments associated with the endeavor.

For decades, Fae has been dealing with dizzy spells, but it's been two years since these have disappeared! Even plantar fasciitis, which had become a pain in the neck for Fae starting in her 50s, also vanished into the blue. It's been years since Fae has been affected by flu and cold-related illnesses. What's more? For years, Fae had borderline high blood pressure. At one point, she went for a blood pressure test, and she got a pleasant surprise—the blood pressure had significantly dropped! Before she started intermittent fasting, Fae had been diagnosed with osteoarthritis, a condition that made climbing up the stairs a difficult task for her. The pain from osteoarthritis gradually decreased until Fae could not feel it anymore. Now, having enjoyed the practical benefits of intermittent fasting, Fae's bet is justified beyond doubt!

Welcome to the 'Revitalize" section, which is represented by the "R" in the GRACE framework. It will specifically discuss the effects of aging and how intermittent fasting addresses them. For instance, aging affects metabolism, hormones, and body functions. In this chapter, we will explore how this happens and how intermittent fasting can be a beneficial tool for aiding hormonal balance, weight management, and improved energy levels as you enjoy your golden years.

THE GOLDEN YEARS: METABOLISM AND HORMONAL SHIFTS

Of course, there are many physical body changes that you might have noticed already. However, did you know that these changes are due to alterations in metabolism, hormones, and other body functions that are relevant for survival? Maybe not, but let's delve more into the nitty-gritty of these changes in this section.

Decreased Metabolic Rate

Metabolism is the process through which your cells use the food that you eat to produce the energy that your body needs for both survival and maintenance. The rate of metabolism is normally high before you reach the age of 20. Once you're beyond 20 years of age, the metabolic rate reduces by 10% after every decade (Piedmont, n.d.). This means that by the time you reach 50 years of age, your metabolism is more likely to be 30% slower. This also translates to the fact that you burn lower amounts of calories as you age, thereby elevating the likelihood of gaining weight, even if you don't increase your food intake. This explains why gaining weight is easier as you age, while shedding extra pounds seems so difficult.

Hormonal Shifts

In women, aging is often accompanied by significant hormonal changes that alter your mood and other bodily functions. By now, you might have already started experiencing these changes and their effects. Hormones are chemicals that are produced by your body and transported to target parts, where they initiate specific functions. Aging can alter the rate at which the hormones are produced, thereby limiting their function and efficacy. In some situations, aging can affect the target organs or tissues so that they become less sensitive to the hormones, even when they are available in the right amounts. Besides, some of the organs that produce certain hormones are regulated by other hormones. This means that any alterations in one hormone may trigger a series of changes in others as well. Imagine the number of hormonal changes that occur under such circumstances.

Let's get more practical. Aging comes with significant fluctuations in estrogen levels. When this happens, you might experience symptoms such as night sweats, reduced libido, hot flashes, fatigue, mood swings, and weight gain. The production of progesterone also drops, causing effects similar to those caused by lower estrogen levels. The human growth hormone is responsible for enhancing your muscle mass, a scenario that increases your energy levels as well. Now, imagine what happens when the production of the hormone reduces, as is the case with women who are aged 50 and above—the muscle mass and energy levels also reduce!

Another hormone that is mainly affected by aging is melatonin, which is usually referred to as the "sleep hormone." This hormone enhances sleep and is produced by your brain when it's dark. This explains why you usually fall asleep at night—interesting, right? However, as you age, less melatonin is produced by your body. As a result, the quality and quantity of your sleep are negatively affected. This may lead to insomnia, a condition that is characterized by inadequate sleep.

Diminished Bone Density

Aging is usually characterized by reduced bone density, irrespective of whether you are male or female. When the loss of bone density is moderate, the condition is referred to as osteopenia, while more severe cases are better described as osteoporosis. After menopause, women are more susceptible to losing their bone density compared to their male counterparts, so the former are more likely to experience osteoporosis. This is because of the lower levels of estrogen during menopause. By the way, estrogen is highly involved in processes that lead to bone formation. Lower estrogen levels weaken your bones, making them more brittle and easier to break.

While estrogen contributes much to reduced bone density, there are more factors involved. As you age, your body's ability to absorb calcium from the food that you eat reduces. You need calcium to make strong bones. However, for your body to effectively use the available calcium, you should have adequate amounts of vitamin D. Unfortunately, the concentration of this vitamin also reduces as the years go by. Therefore, the reduced calcium and vitamin D levels together contribute to reduced strength in your bones.

Please note that the extent to which different bones in your body are affected by aging varies. Some bones are more susceptible to weakening than others. For example, the hip bone easily loses its bone density. The same applies to the bones that are located at the spine and wrists.

Decreased Energy

One of the first noticeable body changes that occurs due to aging is a decrease in basal metabolic rate (BMR). Your BMR is determined by the number of calories that your body burns when you are at rest. This decline in metabolic rate starts at around the age of 30 and then rapidly accelerates after you reach 50. It is partially attributed to reduced muscle mass and changes in hormonal activity. This results in you feeling less energetic, thus needing fewer calories to maintain your weight. Several factors contribute to the decrease in energy that women over 50 experience. A sloweddown metabolism due to reduced muscle mass and hormonal shifts like declining estrogen all play a key role in making you feel less energetic. A drop in estrogen quantities not only affects energy levels but also impacts sleep quality through changes in melatonin, thus further contributing to fatigue. Additionally, the hormonal roller coaster of menopause, coupled with a natural decline in growth hormone, weakens muscles and hinders tissue repair, thereby leaving you feeling less physically capable.

Declined Muscle Mass and Strength

The story doesn't end there. Growth hormone, which is critical for muscle repair and tissue regeneration, also declines steadily with age. This contributes to the loss of muscle mass and reduced strength, which are both often observed in older women. This negatively impacts mobility and physical functions. Additionally, melatonin, the hormone that is responsible for regulating sleep-wake cycles, may decrease, leading to sleep disturbances and daytime fatigue. As you gracefully enter your golden years, other factors also lead to a decline in muscle mass and strength. Hormonal shifts and reduced physical activity are key contributors to this (Hu et al., 2020). The decline in estrogen levels after menopause dampens the process of building and repairing muscle tissue.

This, coupled with a natural decrease in growth hormone, which is another key player in muscle growth and repair, weakens muscles and makes you more susceptible to breakdown. However, there is more to this. Age-related changes in lifestyle often lead to decreased physical activity, thereby further contributing to muscle loss. This inactivity weakens muscles that aren't engaged, thus creating a vicious cycle of decline. But there's hope for you. Understanding these factors empowers you to rewrite your script through regular exercise and a balanced diet, thereby allowing your body to create a balance between hormones, physical activity, and developing stronger muscles.

Changes in Cardiovascular Health

Cardiovascular health also changes as you age. Arteriosclerosis, which is the hardening and thickening of your arteries, becomes more prevalent due to factors like reduced blood flow and increased inflammation. This, along with other changes in blood pressure and cholesterol levels, elevates the risk of heart disease, which is a leading cause of death in women over 50 (Richard, 2018). As you journey into your golden years, your cardiovascular health experiences subtle changes that can be attributed to many factors, like hormonal shifts, arterial stiffening, and changes in blood pressure. The decline in estrogen leads to increased inflammation and a rise in "bad" cholesterol, thereby compromising blood flow and raising the risk of heart disease.

Additionally, your arteries lose their flexibility and become stiffer, making it harder for the heart to pump blood more efficiently. This effect, coupled with increased blood pressure due to factors like stress and weight gain, further strains your cardiovascular system. While this may sound scary, don't be bothered at all. Remember, you are in full control of your dietary choices, and making healthy ones can turn these negative impacts all around! Comprehending these contributing factors empowers you to harmonize your health through lifestyle changes like having a balanced diet and conducting regular body exercises to help manage blood pressure and cholesterol. By taking charge of your eating patterns and physical activities, you can ensure that your cardiovascular system continues to work efficiently throughout your golden years.

Changes in Cognitive Function

Some degree of cognitive decline is inevitable as you age; hence, some brain function changes are quite common. Your brain's processing speed, memory, and executive functions like planning and decision-making may slightly decline. This has been attributed to various factors, including reduced blood flow to the brain, changes in neural composition, and inflammation (Downing, 2022). However, maintaining a healthy lifestyle through regular physical activity, mental stimulation, and consuming a balanced diet can help to mitigate these changes and support cognitive health. While aging doesn't guarantee cognitive decline, women over 50 often experience subtle changes in mental sharpness. Several factors are responsible for this shift. Declining **estrogen** plays a key role in impacting memory and learning potential. Additionally, cognitive function can be affected by reduced blood flow to the brain. Chronic brain inflammation also disrupts normal cognitive function and can contribute to gradual mental decline. Furthermore, other subtle changes in brain structure that come with aging will affect your thoughts and memories and contribute to gradual cognitive decline.

THE SCIENCE BEHIND INTERMITTENT FASTING

As a woman over 50, maneuvering through the complex body changes that you experience during this time can be quite confusing and challenging. However, intermittent fasting offers you a universal remedy for your overall health challenges. This dietary approach, involving cycles of eating and fasting, holds many health benefits that resonate with the specific concerns of this age group through its alternating eating and fasting cycles. Intermittent fasting can help boost the decline in metabolism that is common after 50, thereby reducing oxidative stress in your body and triggering cellular repair mechanisms.

According to research, intermittent fasting can also improve insulin sensitivity, thereby indirectly supporting bone mineral density (Johns Hopkins Medicine, 2021). If you are feeling the effects of hormonal shifts on your cardiovascular health, then intermittent fasting might help you by reducing inflammation and improving blood sugar control, thereby lowering your risk of heart disease. You can also enjoy excellent brain health through engaging in the practice, with research suggesting that improved cognitive function and mental clarity occur during fasting periods. Combining intermittent fasting with a balanced diet and maintaining a healthy lifestyle will enable you to be in control of your well-being and create a healthier and more vibrant aging chapter in your life.

Weight Reduction Through Intermittent Fasting

For women over 50, the incessant whispers of aging characterized by weight gain can tarnish your golden years. However, all these concerns about weight gain can be put to rest by practicing intermittent fasting. This dietary approach taps into your body's natural ability to burn fat more efficiently, thus contributing to significant weight reduction. Intermittent fasting has been shown to boost the aspects of metabolism that promote your body's ability to burn excess fat. By strategically cycling between your eating and fasting periods, you can effectively influence how your body utilizes its energy. During fasting, your body starts to tap into stored fat reserves for fuel, potentially leading to weight loss. Additionally, intermittent fasting is thought to improve insulin sensitivity, which can further assist in regulating blood sugar and promoting healthy weight management for women over 50.

Enhanced Hormonal Balance Through Intermittent Fasting

When it comes to your body, hormones play an instrumental role in influencing everything, from your energy levels to your mood. Intermittent fasting, with its cycles of eating and fasting, can shift your hormonal balance in ways that benefit your health. Let's explore some of the positive changes that this practice can bring to your health:

- **Decreased insulin levels:** Insulin is the hormone that is commonly associated with blood sugar regulation. It takes center stage during the periods after food consumption. However, its role changes during your fast. With no incoming sugars, insulin steps back, thereby allowing your body to access alternative fuel sources that are stored as fat. This radical shift allows for more efficient fat-burning and improved insulin sensitivity in the long run.
- **Enhanced human growth hormone (HGH) levels:** This is a hormone that is responsible for cell repair and tissue regeneration. This hormone plays a very minor role in your body under normal circumstances. However, during a fasting period, the activities of HGH become more

prominent. Its levels increase significantly, such that the hormone begins to support muscle growth, bone density, and even cognitive function.

- **Increased norepinephrine:** Norepinephrine is the hormone that is often associated with the "fight-or-flight" response in your body. However, during a fast, its increased levels play a supportive role in your overall health. Norepinephrine helps to mobilize stored body fat, thereby making it more readily available as fuel for energy and boosting your metabolic rate (Gunnars, 2021). This addition to your hormonal balance promotes efficient energy utilization throughout your fasting period.

These are just a few of the hormonal shifts that are orchestrated by intermittent fasting. Once you begin the practice, you will experience even more of these merits personally. While individual experiences may vary, understanding intermittent fasting's overall positive changes that are brought about by inducing endocrine shifts allows you to harmonize your body's activities with these hormonal changes.

Increased Energy Levels Through Intermittent Fasting

As you are approaching the end of a fasting window, your body undergoes a remarkable transformation. During this time, your metabolism, which usually operates at a steady tempo, receives a massive jolt of energy. Studies suggest that intermittent fasting, particularly time-restricted feeding within an eight-hour window, can boost your metabolic rate (Li et al., 2021). Research also indicates an increase in calorie burning during fasting periods, which is most likely due to changes in hormones like norepinephrine and the human growth hormone. Norepinephrine mobilizes your fat stores for fuel, while the human growth hormone promotes muscle repair, thereby preventing metabolic slowdown.

Also, time-restricted feeding within an eight-hour window specifically holds unique benefits for women over 50, since this schedule positively impacts reproductive hormone levels. Studies suggest that it may improve insulin sensitivity, thereby indirectly supporting bone mineral density, which is a concern that is often linked to declining estrogen (Li et al., 2021). Additionally, early research also indicates reduced levels of inflammatory markers and improved blood sugar control through intermittent fasting, thus lowering the risk of heart disease, which is a common concern in this age group.

ACHIEVING HORMONAL HARMONY THROUGH INTERMITTENT FASTING

Intermittent fasting can help you achieve hormonal balance much easier. Let's go deeper into how it impacts three major hormones in your body:

Insulin

Insulin facilitates the movement of sugar from the bloodstream into cells. During periods of constant eating, this hormone is constantly active. This can lead to potential hormonal imbalances. When you begin intermittent fasting, the action of insulin decreases due to reduced food intake. This shift allows your body to switch fuel sources, and your metabolism begins burning stored fat instead of relying solely on incoming sugars. The result is improved insulin sensitivity, with cells responding more effectively to insulin signals. This reduced insulin resistance can lower your risk of developing or aggravating type 2 diabetes by facilitating better blood sugar management (DeCesaris, 2023). Think of this as a preventive measure that ensures that your metabolism doesn't get overwhelmed by the constant influx of sugars.

Ghrelin

Ghrelin, which is also known as the hunger hormone, plays a vital role in your appetite. It constantly reminds you to eat. During extended periods of fasting, ghrelin release initially rises, leading to hunger pangs. However, as your fasting progresses, the ghrelin levels begin to gradually decline. This shift leads to reduced hunger and increased feelings of satiety (DeCesaris, 2023). You might be surprised by how easily you can manage extended fasting periods without constant cravings. This is the result of Ghrelin's action. This hormonal change promotes sustainable eating patterns, which help you stay in control of your calorie intake. This allows you to achieve your health goals through intermittent fasting much easier.

Leptin

Leptin is often referred to as the satiety hormone and plays a crucial role in appetite regulation. This hormone is responsible for reminding you to stop eating when you're full. During a fast, leptin levels initially decrease, mimicking the hunger sensations triggered by ghrelin. However, as your fast progresses and your body taps into stored fat reserves, leptin levels begin to rise. This increase sends a powerful signal of fullness, explaining why you might not feel like eating a few hours after starting your fast. This improved leptin sensitivity promotes effortless food portion control and prevents overeating, thereby helping you maintain a healthy weight and energy balance (Cienfuegos et al., 2022).

COGNITIVE BENEFITS OF INTERMITTENT FASTING

While the benefits of intermittent fasting often focus on physical health, its impact on your mind is nothing short of remarkable. Your brain is responsible for memory, focus, and emotional well-being. Intermittent fasting coordinates your brain's performance, leading to benefits such as:

- **Improved mental function:** According to research findings, intermittent fasting can be a powerful tool for enhancing mental function (Gunnars, 2021). During fasting periods, the brain shifts its fuel source from readily available glucose to ketones, produced from stored fat. This metabolic switch leads to increased neuroplasticity. Neuroplasticity refers to your brain's capacity to reorganize itself by forming new neural connections. This translates to improved memory, faster processing speed, and sharper focus, allowing you to tackle tasks with renewed alertness and mental agility.
- **Increased neurogenesis:** This process is characterized by the sprouting of new neurons inside your brain. Studies show that neurogenesis can be triggered by intermittent fasting (Gunnars, 2021). This increase in neuronal growth, particularly in the hippocampus, a region that is crucial for learning and memory, can bolster cognitive function and is thought to protect against age-related cognitive decline. This ultimately allows for richer thought and creativity.
- **Reduced anxiety and improved mood:** Stress and anxiety disrupt your emotions, leading to negative feelings and reduced mental clarity. However, intermittent fasting can play a calming role, according to research evidence on the practice (Gunnars, 2021). By reducing inflammation and lowering stress hormones like cortisol, intermittent fasting

can help improve your mood and anxiety levels. This emotional balance is achieved through hormonal shifts and allows for clearer thinking. This, in turn, promotes a sense of well-being, which allows you to experience your life with greater emotional composure.

- **Enhanced mental clarity:** The combined effects of enhanced neurogenesis, improved cognitive function, and better mood culminate in improved mental clarity. Experiencing sharper focus, improved memory, and a calmer emotional state allows you to go through your daily life routines with renewed confidence and mental energy. This state of mental clarity can be achieved by practicing intermittent fasting, thereby empowering you to think, feel, and experience life to the fullest.

You learned the impact of intermittent fasting on your metabolism, specifically how the practice impacts your hormones, in this chapter. Hormonal shifts in estrogen, progesterone, and the human growth hormone, that occur during and after menopause cause several physical issues. These can be remediated by intermittent fasting, as it brings these hormones back into balance. Practicing intermittent fasting might seem daunting at first, but the practice gradually becomes manageable as your body gets used to it. With the right knowledge and guidance, you can choose the best intermittent fasting method that suits your preferences, lifestyle, and body's needs. In the next chapter, I will take you through different intermittent fasting approaches that you may consider. Come along.

GETTING STARTED WITH INTERMITTENT FASTING

At 68, Seralisa had battled weight issues for decades and tried every fad diet and exercise program. Twelve years ago, the slightest hunger pangs would have triggered frantic attempts to pull out a small bite or little sip from her fridge. This made the guilt-laden echoes of overeating repeatedly ring in Seralisa's ears. When she stumbled upon intermittent fasting, the seemingly simple approach guided her toward an almost immediate transformation to excellent well-being. Her body quickly adapted to the practice, and she began enjoying sustained energy and significant weight loss. But the benefits went far beyond her physical body. Her brain fog slowly gave way to a sharp focus that even took her by surprise, as it came just as fast. Her mood also significantly improved. Additionally, she discovered a new love for active body movements through aerobics, as her body no longer felt like the burden it was before.

Chelsea, 59, was now fed up with always feeling exhausted. The fatigue drained away her energy and enthusiasm. Despite a healthy diet and regular exercise, the spark for these activities seemed to have been lost. Then one day, she came across intermittent fasting. Her body's initial adjustment to the routine was bumpy, but soon, she began to experience remarkable changes. Tasks that once felt challenging became more manageable, and the fatigue began to slowly loosen its grip, replaced by a surge of revitalized energy. Intrigued by her transformation, Chelsea became even more eager to understand the science behind this powerful dietary tool. This exploration led her down a fascinating path that uncovered a multitude of other intermittent fasting techniques, each with its own unique approach. Join me in this chapter as I unveil some of these diverse strategies that you can adopt for your intermittent fast. This chapter will also empower you to discover the unique fasting approach that resonates with your body, lifestyle, and preferences. It tackles the "A" in the GRACE acronym, standing for "adaptation," whose essence is to guide you through the initial steps of intermittent fasting.

SUITABLE INTERMITTENT FASTING METHODS FOR WOMEN OVER 50

Your golden years shimmer with promise, but the reality of your body's changes can make everything feel more discordant. As a woman over 50, aspects such as shifting hormones, changing metabolism, and gradually diminishing energy levels may be inevitable. The different rhythms for intermittent fasting that exist within this dietary approach make it necessary for you to find the right one that empowers you for a healthier and more vibrant future. Let's explore these different fasting approaches together to help you discover the one that resonates with your body and unlocks a beautiful composition and excellent well-being.

The 16:8 Method (Daily Fasting Plan)

If you are seeking a gentle introduction to intermittent fasting, the 16:8 method, also known as daily fasting, might be the perfect way to begin. It allows you to eat throughout an eight-hour window, leaving 16 hours for your body to rest and reset.

- **Advantages**: This flexible approach easily integrates into your normal daily routines by allowing you to choose an eight-hour eating window that suits your lifestyle. This could mean enjoying an early dinner. Studies suggest improved metabolism, weight loss, and even enhanced cognitive function are the benefits of conducting this fast (Gunnars, 2020).
- **Considerations**: During your eating window, remember to prioritize a balanced diet that is rich in fruits, vegetables, and whole grains to nourish your body. Also, be mindful of staying hydrated throughout your fast. With its simplicity and health benefits, the 16:8 method is ideally the first harmonious fasting approach that you may consider beginning with.

12-Hour or Overnight Fasting

If you are seeking a natural rhythm to your fasting journey as a woman over 50, then the 12-hour or overnight method might be a good choice. This fasting approach mimics your body's natural sleep-wake cycle. This 12-hour window, stretching from dinner to breakfast, resonates with your body's circadian rhythm, thereby making it easier to follow and integrate into your daily routine.

- **Advantages**: Research indicates improved insulin sensitivity, thereby possibly reducing the risk of diabetes, and the potential to manage weight effectively (WebMD Editorial Contributors, 2021). However, remember that discipline in keeping up with this routine is essential.
- **Considerations**: Resist the urge to snack after dinner so that you can allow your body to truly rest and reset during the fasting window. While this method might not be as dramatic for significant weight loss compared to others, its alignment with your natural rhythm and its health benefits make it a compelling option.

14:10 Fasting

The 14:10 method offers a middle ground if you are seeking a balance between fasting benefits and lifestyle flexibility. This method is characterized by 14 hours of rest from eating, followed by a 10-hour feasting window. The 14:10 approach allows you to experience the benefits of fasting without drastically shifting your eating habits. Whether you prefer an extended morning fast or a longer period without eating, after having an early dinner, the 14:10 method lets you choose a rhythm that sits comfortably with you.

- **Advantages**: This method can aid in weight management and improve your metabolic health, although its benefits might be less pronounced compared to longer fasting periods.
- **Considerations**: Remember, the key to maintaining a healthy diet during your eating window lies in adjusting meal times whenever necessary. If longer fasts seem daunting, the 14:10 method might be a manageable first step in your fasting journey.

Eat Stop Eat Approach

The Eat Stop Eat method offers you a bold 24-hour fast twice a week. This approach promises weight loss and metabolic health improvements. You devote two days solely to internal cleansing, followed by five days of healthy nourishment. The Eat Stop Eat method, unlike other daily routines, requires commitment only on specific days, thereby offering flexibility for busy schedules.

- **Advantages**: This approach has been proven to bring metabolic benefits like reduced inflammation and enhanced insulin sensitivity, while also ensuring remarkable weight loss (Stanton, 2021).
- **Considerations**: Sustaining such long fasts can be difficult, and the risk of overindulging on non-fasting days is real. Additionally, seeing results might take longer compared to more frequent fasting schedules. Weigh these considerations carefully and make professional medical consultations before beginning this transformative, yet demanding, approach. If you seek significant change and thrive on overcoming challenges, then the Eat Stop Eat method might be a powerful option to consider.

The 5:2 Intermittent Fasting Method

This approach is flexible and easier to incorporate. The 5:2 method allows you to enjoy your regular eating habits for five days, and then dedicate two non-consecutive days to a lower-calorie intake of around 500–600 calories. With this approach, you can enjoy the delights of normal eating for most of the week, making it more sustainable than daily fasting methods.

- **Advantages**: The benefits of this approach go beyond weight management to include improved metabolism, reduced inflammation, and even a lower risk of developing chronic diseases like heart disease and type 2 diabetes (Gunnars, 2020). However, remember that those two low-calorie days are still part of the dietary routine, so you need to remain disciplined throughout.
- **Considerations**: While 500–600 calories are generally recommended, individual needs may vary. Consulting a dietary professional beforehand ensures that your nutritional needs are met even on fasting days. Additionally, some people might find the calorie restriction challenging, so it is important to regularly adjust your approach based on your body's response to intermittent fasting.

Alternate Day Fasting (ADF)

Alternate-day fasting is a powerful but demanding dietary approach. It offers a sharp contrast between feasting and fasting. This method alternates your full days of fasting, whereby you consume only water, black coffee, or unsweetened tea, with regular eating days.

- **Advantages**: Research has shown encouraging results like metabolic health improvements, including reduced inflammation and increased insulin sensitivity, through this fasting approach. Significant weight loss has also been reported (Al Qudsi, 2022).
- **Considerations**: Remember that this demanding fasting rhythm isn't for everyone. Sticking to full fasting days can be challenging, and possible side effects like fatigue and irritability might occur. Additionally, ensuring adequate

nutrient intake on eating days is crucial. If you have underlying health conditions, I recommend you consult your healthcare professional before considering ADF.

24-Hour Fasts

The 24-hour fast, where you abstain from food from dinner one day to dinner the next, offers a potent dietary option for women over 50 if you are seeking significant weight loss.

- **Advantages**: The 24-hour pause in your usual eating rhythm allows your body to reset and focus on internal cleansing. Practiced once or twice a week, this approach can lead to substantial calorie reduction, thereby promoting faster weight loss compared to other approaches.
- **Considerations**: This extended fast can trigger more rapid muscle breakdown, considering that muscle mass naturally declines with age. Muscle loss can negatively impact metabolism and long-term health. It is crucial to have professional medical consultations before embarking on this demanding approach to ensure its safety and effectiveness.

FASTING STYLES

Approaching intermittent fasting without considering your unique composition can lead to disharmony. Here are key factors to consider before embarking on this journey:

- **Health status:** Start by paying attention to your body's unique needs. Healthcare consultation is paramount in cases of preexisting health issues like diabetes, heart disease, or kidney issues, as certain fasting methods might not be suitable for you.

- **Lifestyle and schedule:** Before you begin your intermittent fasting journey, carefully consider your daily rhythm. Are you an early bird or a night owl? Do you work long hours or have unpredictable routines? Choose a fasting plan that integrates seamlessly into your lifestyle, like the 16:8 method for flexible fasting windows or the 5:2 approach for normal eating most days.

- **Dietary preferences:** Are you a meat-eater, a vegetarian, or somewhere in between? Explore fasting methods that complement your dietary choices. Healthy eating should always be the foundation, regardless of your chosen fasting approach.

- **Experience with fasting:** Are you a beginner or a seasoned faster? If you're new to fasting, start with gentler methods like the 12-hour or 5:2 plans. Gradually increase the intensity as your body adapts.

- **Weight loss goals:** While fasting can aid weight management, don't make it your sole focus. Consider your overall health and choose a plan that supports sustainable weight loss, like the Eat Stop Eat, or Alternate Day Fasting for more significant calorie reduction.

- **Metabolic health:** Fasting's impact on metabolism varies depending on the method and your health. If you have concerns about insulin sensitivity or other metabolic factors, discuss them with a healthcare professional and choose a plan with potential metabolic benefits like the 16:8 or 12-hour approach.

The ideal fasting plan is a combination of the factors highlighted above. Remain attentive to your body's cues by exploring and experimenting with different combinations of factors. With this mindful approach, you can turn fasting into an effective dietary instrument for ensuring your overall well-being.

Matching Fasting Styles to Individual Needs

Always remember that fasting isn't a one-size-fits-all approach, but an approach that is conducted to suit your unique individual needs. Here's how to match some common profiles with the right fasting approach:

- **The beginner:** Stepping into the world of intermittent fasting can feel daunting. Thus, the 12:12 method offers a much gentler introduction. This approach requires you to simply shift your usual eating window by a few hours, fast for 12 hours, and eat within a 12-hour period. With this method, you could decide to postpone breakfast or enjoy an early dinner. This seemingly small change in your feeding schedule has significant benefits. Start slow and gradually progress to explore other methods as you become more comfortable, while carefully observing your body's response to the practice.
- **The busy professional:** Strict deadlines and schedules may make it difficult for you to engage in intermittent fasting. However, with the 16:8 method, it is easier to incorporate this practice into your day. The flexibility of this method lies in choosing an eight-hour window that suits your schedule.
- **The health-conscious dieter:** Weight management is important, but so is overall health. The 5:2 diet harmonizes both concerns. This approach lets you enjoy five days of your regular eating habits, and then you reduce your calorie intake to between 500 and 600 calories on two non-consecutive days. Think of it as a mindful

reset, which focuses on nutrient-rich dietary choices on your low-calorie days. This dietary approach isn't about food restriction but about mindful eating and promoting healthy habits for long-term well-being.

- **The experienced faster:** If you've explored the initial fasting methods and are ready for a more complex approach, alternate-day fasting can challenge your body and accelerate your progress. This method demands that you attend to your body closely and commit deeply to the routine. Get a detailed assessment before embarking on this rigorous approach, should you have any prior health concerns. Remember to ensure adequate nutrition on eating days and be aware of possible drawbacks like fatigue and irritability.

GUIDELINES FOR SAFELY STARTING INTERMITTENT FASTING

Embarking on intermittent fasting requires adequate physical and mental preparation. Do not allow your body to dive into this practice unprepared. Remember, proper preparation will help you avoid uncomfortable side effects and enjoy the full potential of this powerful health tool.

Mental Preparation

Do not allow your mind to approach intermittent fasting haphazardly. Here are some key mental preparations to ensure a successful fasting experience:

- **Educate yourself:** Understanding the "why" behind your efforts is essential when conducting your fast. Immerse yourself in credible educational resources, consult healthcare professionals, and learn enough about different fasting methods and their potential benefits and drawbacks. This empowers you to make informed choices and adapt any approach to your unique needs.

- **Set clear goals:** Don't begin a fasting approach simply because it's trending. Instead, clearly define your personal goals, be they weight management, improved energy, or metabolic health. Aligning your fasting practice with clear, achievable goals keeps you motivated and provides a guiding light throughout the process.
- **Cultivate self-love and mindfulness:** Your fast is not about restriction or punishing yourself. Rather, it's about nurturing your body with mindful choices. During your eating window, embrace self-love by focusing on keeping your body nourished with healthy foods. Practice mindfulness by tuning into your hunger cues and honoring your body's signals.
- **Manage expectations:** Don't fall prey to quick-fix promises or unrealistic expectations. Fasting is a sustainable lifestyle shift, not a magic bullet. Set realistic expectations about achievable progress and celebrate small victories along the way, focusing on long-term well-being over immediate results.
- **Prepare for challenges:** Like any worthwhile endeavor, fasting comes with its fair share of challenges. Be prepared for initial hunger pangs, mood swings, and changes in energy levels. Acknowledge these as temporary hurdles, not permanent roadblocks. Develop coping mechanisms like healthy snacking, stress management techniques, and a strong, supportive network of people to help you overcome these challenges effectively.

Physical Preparation

Your physical well-being demands adequate preparation for optimal results. Here are some crucial steps to set yourself up for a rewarding fasting experience:

- **Get a prior health assessment:** This is paramount, especially in cases of preexisting medical concerns like diabetes, heart disease, or kidney issues. Your healthcare professional can assess your suitability for fasting, address any concerns, and align you with healthy and effective methods according to your unique health profile.
- **Start slow:** Don't jump into extended fasts immediately. Ease into the rhythm by starting with shorter fasting windows, like the 12:12 method. Gradually increase the duration as your body adapts.
- **Prioritize nutrition:** Fasting doesn't mean neglecting healthy eating. During your eating window, focus on nourishing your body with nutrient-rich whole foods like vegetables, fruits, healthy fats, and lean proteins. This ensures that your body receives the essential vitamins, minerals, and macronutrients it needs to function optimally during your fasting periods.
- **Stay hydrated:** Regardless of your fasting window, strive to stay hydrated during the day. Staying hydrated helps with detoxification, regulates body temperature, and supports various bodily functions, ensuring smooth operation during fasting periods.
- **Incorporate resistance training:** Although it may initially be tempting to focus solely on cardio, don't neglect resistance training. Building and maintaining muscle mass is crucial for metabolic health and long-term weight management. Incorporate strength training exercises into

your fasting routine, even if it's just bodyweight exercises at home, to counteract the possible muscle loss that you may experience and maximize the benefits of fasting.

Starting an Intermittent Fasting Routine

If you are ready to embark on the stimulating journey of intermittent fasting, it is important to remember that a mindful approach paves the way for sustainable success. Here's a step-by-step guide to managing your initial fasting days safely and effectively:

- **Choose a fasting plan and schedule your meals:** Research different fasting methods and explore options like the 16:8, 5:2, or Eat Stop Eat methods. You may also discuss the suitability of these approaches with a healthcare professional. Choose a plan that integrates seamlessly into your schedule.
- **Ease into fasting:** Shorter fasting windows are ideal for beginners. Start with the 12:12 method, before progressing to longer fasts. If you experience intense hunger, headaches, or dizziness, take appropriate actions such as hydrating yourself, eating balanced meals, and resting. Consider avoiding any strenuous activities until you've fully recovered. You might even need to review your intermittent fasting method so that you go for a milder one. If symptoms persist or get more severe, be sure to consult with a healthcare professional.
- **Monitor your body's response:** Regularly monitor your energy levels, sleep quality, and any changes in mood or digestion. If you experience any unpleasant side effects, shorten your fasting window, or modify your plan. Also, be sure to acknowledge and celebrate positive changes to keep you motivated on your journey.

- **Stay active:** Include moderate-intensity exercises like cycling, swimming, or brisk walking. Be attentive to your body, while adjusting your workout intensity based on your energy levels during fasting. Remember to choose activities you enjoy to keep you active. Exercise should be sustainable, so find something that you truly love to do, and avoid strenuous physical activity, especially during longer fasts. If you feel overly tired, prioritize rest, and reschedule your workout.

- **Hydrate and replenish electrolytes:** Keep yourself adequately hydrated. Each day, aim for between eight and ten glasses of water, and even more during longer fasts. Also, consider including natural electrolytes like coconut water, herbal teas, or broth in your diet, especially during extended fasts.

- **Regularly assess your progress:** Track your body changes over time, but keep in mind that weight isn't the sole measure of success during intermittent fasting. Evaluate your overall well-being by considering improvements in energy levels, sleep quality, and digestion. Avoid obsessing over short-term results, but rather focus on sustainable changes and long-term well-being. Also, avoid comparing yourself to others. Progress is individual; therefore, celebrate your achievements.

- **Attend to your body's cues and maintain consistency:** Respect your hunger signals and break your fast if you feel excessively hungry or unwell. Regularly modify your fasting plan based on your body's needs.

Intermittent Fasting Guidelines

While complete abstinence is the hallmark of a true fast, remember that some things are still allowed during your fasting window. Most importantly, focus intently on adequately hydrating yourself by sipping on water, unsweetened tea, or black coffee throughout your fasting period. For added electrolytes, consider organic options like bone broth or coconut water. If your chosen fasting method allows, small amounts of healthy fats like medium-chain triglyceride (MCT) oil or a splash of milk in your coffee can help manage your hunger pangs. Remember to stick to zero-calorie options and avoid sugary drinks, artificial sweeteners, or any food that triggers a significant insulin response, as this can break your fast. Remember, the goal is to let your body rest and reset, so prioritize clean hydration and pay regular attention to how you are adjusting, to make the most of your fasting experience.

Tips for Integrating Fasting Into Daily Routines

Integrating fasting into your daily routine should blend smoothly with your life's rhythm. Aim for progress, not perfection. Choose a fasting plan that complements your schedule and preferences, and avoid working against them. Remember, flexibility is key to your fasting approach, in addition to these other considerations:

- **Setting realistic goals:** Start small and begin with shorter fasting windows, like 12-hour durations. As your body adjusts, gradually increase the duration. Remember to focus on progress and consistency, not perfection. Occasional "off days" won't derail your progress. Along the way, also remember to celebrate improvements in energy levels, focus, or sleep quality, not just weight loss.

- **Selecting the right fasting plan:** Do your research properly prior to beginning fasting and choose one that fits your lifestyle and preferences. Constantly adjust your fasting window based on your body's response as you go. Additionally, get professional guidance on the plan that is best suited for your health issues and individual needs.
- **Managing social situations:** Learn to communicate openly. Inform your friends and family about your fasting practice and politely decline meals or explain alternative options. Engage in conversations and other unrelated activities during social gatherings instead of focusing solely on food. You may also offer to bring a dish that you can enjoy without compromising on your fasting goals.
- **Staying consistent:** Always prepare your snacks and meals beforehand. Prepare healthy options in advance to avoid unhealthy choices during hunger attacks. Finding an accountability partner will also help to keep you in check. Having someone share your goals and challenges provides support and motivation to keep you aligned with your fasting goals.

This chapter has taken you through the different intermittent fasting approaches that you can consider for your fast. These approaches include the common 12:12 method, which is suitable for beginners, and the slightly more complex 16:8 approach, which suits you better if you have a busier schedule or have somewhat gotten used to intermittent fasting. Before beginning any fasting approach, it is crucial to professionally evaluate your health. This chapter also details the importance of physical and mental preparation before you begin intermittent fasting. This facilitates easier body adjustments to the practice once you begin. Tips on integrating intermittent fasting into your daily routine were also shared with you, including selecting the right fasting plan and staying consistent with the practice. As you follow these guidelines, your mental clarity and energy levels will be naturally boosted. Follow me into the next chapter for more on this.

POWERING UP YOUR ENERGY LEVELS AND MENTAL CLARITY

Karyn Shank, a practicing medical physician, always preached healthy living. Yet, beneath her confident exterior, fatigue lurked. Her vegetarian, low-fat diet left her craving for more food, and the stress of managing her practice gradually sapped her energy away. Sleep was elusive, and finding joy felt like an uphill battle. One day, a patient introduced her to intermittent fasting. Skeptical but intrigued, Karyn embarked on a 16:8 journey. She found it challenging to adjust to the schedule in the beginning. Her stomach constantly grumbled, and old habits of irresponsible eating were a persistent temptation. But slowly, a positive shift began. The afternoon slump vanished, replaced by sustained energy that lasted her throughout the day. Her mind also became more clear and sharper. Karyn was surprised by intermittent fasting's impact on her energy and focus. She rediscovered the joy of cooking while experimenting with healthy and satisfying meals during her eating window. The guilt of occasional treats gradually subsided and was replaced by a balanced approach to eating.

However, the positive changes that Karyn experienced weren't just physical. Once easily provoked and prone to stress, she found a newfound resilience against mental instability and became much calmer. The mental clarity translated into sharper problem-solving and a renewed curiosity for her medical practice. Long-lost laughter became a testament to the joy that had found its way back into Karyn's life. She felt lighter, not just in weight, but also in spirit. Karyn's story is about rediscovering physical and mental energy and is proof of the importance of assessing your body to find a personalized approach to intermittent fasting. Karyn, who was once an exhausted doctor, now stands as a beacon of vitality. Her story is a powerful reminder that you, too, can power up your energy levels and mental clarity through intermittent fasting. I will take you through the relationship between intermittent fasting, improved energy levels, and mental clarity in this chapter. The chapter explores the "C" of the GRACE framework, which is culti-vation, thus providing strategies for you to feel more energized during your fast. Let's continue reading.

THE PSYCHOLOGICAL RELATIONSHIP BETWEEN INTERMITTENT FASTING, ENERGY LEVELS, AND MENTAL CLARITY

Your body is just like a busy workstation, where energy flows constantly, and mental clarity is one of the immediate results of this. Intermittent fasting harmonizes the essential metabolic elements that allow for swift positive changes in your body. Now, you may be curious about the process and how it unfolds. Well, to break it down in a very simple way, your body enters a state of fuel switching during a fast. Initially, your body burns through the readily available glucose from your meals. But once that source is depleted, it taps into ketone bodies for energy. Ketone bodies are an alternative fuel that is produced by the liver from stored fat.

This switch is very important. Ketones offer a cleaner and more efficient burning of energy stores by reducing the burden on your digestive system and pancreas (Johns Hopkins Medicine, 2021). Thus, they allow your body to shift to a cleaner and more sustainable energy source.

This metabolic shift also triggers a cascade of hormonal changes. Insulin levels drop, thereby promoting fat burning and cellular repair. Conversely, glucagon levels rise, thus signaling your body to release stored glucose for immediate needs. This hormonal change improves your insulin sensitivity, which in turn prevents those dreaded energy crashes and promotes sustained energy throughout the day. But the positive transformations of intermittent fasting don't stop there. This practice also impacts the brain-derived neurotrophic factor (BDNF) in your body. BDNF is a vital protein that helps to generate new brain neurons and boost neuroplasticity (Gunnars, 2021). Neuroplasticity is the brain's ability to reorganize itself by forming new neuron connections. This translates to sharper mental focus, improved memory, and even boosted creativity. Intermittent fasting can also reduce inflammation, which is an undesirable condition that is linked to fatigue and brain fog. By quieting your body's inflammatory noise, intermittent fasting helps to create a clearer mental state, which allows you to think and process information with greater ease.

INTERMITTENT FASTING AND METABOLISM, BRAIN FUNCTION, AND OVERALL COGNITIVE PERFORMANCE

Intermittent fasting has, in recent times, slowly established itself as a useful practice for improving not just body composition but also cognitive function and overall well-being. While further research is still needed, current studies suggest promising benefits for metabolism, brain health, and cognitive performance. Here's an insightful look into some of the beneficial mechanisms that are induced by intermittent fasting:

How Intermittent Fasting Improves Your Metabolism

While weight loss often goes hand-in-hand with intermittent fasting, its benefits go beyond the scale. Studies suggest that this practice boosts your metabolism, thereby leading to more efficient calorie burning and improved overall health (Johns Hopkins Medicine, 2021). Some of the metabolic functions include:

- **Fuel switching:** During fasting, your body transitions from burning the readily available glucose to utilizing fat stores for energy. This "fuel switching" stimulates the production of ketone bodies, which are an alternative fuel source that efficiently fuels the brain and other organs. Additionally, it increases fat oxidation, which allows the body to tap into stored fat for energy, thereby leading to potential weight loss and improved metabolic health.
- **Hormonal balance:** Intermittent fasting influences the balance of key hormones like insulin and glucagon in your body. Lower insulin levels promote fat burning and cellular repair, while increased glucagon levels mobilize stored glucose for immediate needs. This hormonal equilibrium improves insulin sensitivity, thus preventing energy crashes and supporting sustained energy levels.

How Intermittent Fasting Improves Brain Function

Intermittent fasting impacts your brain in the following ways:

- **Neurotrophic factor boost:** The levels of BDNF in your body are naturally boosted by intermittent fasting. BDNF is your body's neurotrophic factor, and its boosting translates to enhanced memory, learning, and heightened creativity. This action is synonymous with fine-tuning your brain for better information processing and cognitive flexibility.
- **Inflammation reduction:** Chronic inflammation can impair brain function and contribute to cognitive decline. Research confirms that brain and body inflammation can be reduced by intermittent fasting, thereby leading you to experience much clearer mental pictures. This clears away mental cloudiness and allows your brain to operate at its best (Santosh Yoga Institute, 2023).
- **Increased cellular energy:** When your brain cells receive a stable and efficient energy source like ketones, they function more optimally. This leads to improved focus, concentration, and mental clarity.

Intermittent Fasting and Overall Cognitive Performance

Your overall cognitive performance is enhanced by intermittent fasting in the following ways:

- **Enhanced memory and learning:** Studies have established that memory consolidation and spatial learning in both animals and humans can be enhanced by practicing intermittent fasting. This is thought to be due to increased BDNF levels and improved communication between brain cells (Santosh Yoga Institute, 2023).

- **Mood and well-being:** Some studies have found intermittent fasting to improve mood and reduce the symptoms of depression and anxiety. The mechanisms behind this phenomenon are still being explored, but the positive outcome includes reduced inflammation, altered neurotransmitter levels, and improved sleep quality (Wang & Wu, 2022).
- **Neuroprotection:** Intermittent fasting may offer neuroprotective benefits, thereby reducing the risk of neurodegenerative diseases like Alzheimer's and Parkinson's, as reported by numerous studies (Wang & Wu, 2022).

Do note, however, that not everyone will enjoy the positive results of intermittent fasting. Get professional medical advice before starting the practice, and keep listening to how your body responds to the fast. Also, be sure to combine intermittent fasting with a healthy diet, adequate sleep, and regular exercise for optimal results. Remember to stay informed about the latest findings on the practice and approach it with healthy mindfulness and individual awareness.

RESEARCH AND RELEVANT STUDIES SUPPORTING THE CONNECTION BETWEEN INTERMITTENT FASTING, ENERGY LEVELS, AND MENTAL CLARITY

The potential of intermittent fasting to impact energy levels and mental clarity has provoked the interest of researchers and individuals alike. To fully understand the mechanisms at play in the practice, more research is still needed. However, several current studies shed encouraging reviews:

- **Journal of clinical nutrition study:** This study explored the combined effects of continuous energy restriction, intermittent fasting, and exercise on factors that influence energy levels and mood. The study involved several obese and overweight adults who participated in either intermittent fasting or structured calorie reduction with or without exercise for 12 weeks. Interestingly, the researchers found that physical exercise conducted with both structured calorie restriction and intermittent fasting led to significant improvements in dietary compliance, perceived hunger, and mood. This suggests that intermittent fasting, when paired with exercise, may help individuals manage hunger and maintain dietary adherence, thus contributing to sustained energy levels and a more positive outlook (Keenan et al., 2022).
- **Annual review of nutrition study:** This comprehensive review analyzed multiple studies on the impact of different fasting methods on weight, metabolism, and related factors. The review confirmed that all forms of food restriction practices, including intermittent fasting, resulted in mild to moderate weight loss, which can positively influence energy levels. The review also highlighted the interesting finding that many individuals experience "dietary euphoria" on fasting days, reporting increased energy and improved mood. This suggests that the metabolic shifts that are triggered by intermittent fasting directly impact energy levels and cognitive function (University of Illinois, 2021).

UNDERSTANDING THE RELEVANCE OF THE RESEARCH FINDINGS ON INTERMITTENT FASTING

The Journal of Clinical Nutrition's study emphasizes the prospective cooperation between intermittent fasting, exercise, and dietary adherence in managing hunger and mood. These are factors that can significantly impact your energy levels. The research findings suggest that a holistic approach that incorporates other dietary interventions might be more effective than simply relying on intermittent fasting alone. The Annual Review of Nutrition's study points toward the weight-loss aspect of fasting and its potential connection to increased energy. However, the research also acknowledges the intriguing phenomenon of "fasting euphoria," suggesting that there might be more direct metabolic and neurological mechanisms at play during intermittent fasting, beyond just weight loss.

The research studies also highlighted that individual responses to intermittent fasting can vary significantly. This necessitates a full medical review to assess your body's suitability for the practice before commencing the practice and then tailoring the approach to suit your body's unique needs. While encouraging, these studies don't conclusively prove a cause-and-effect relationship between intermittent fasting and enhanced energy levels or mental clarity. Further research is thus needed to fully understand the biological mechanisms that are triggered by intermittent fasting and its long-term implications for your body.

STRATEGIES FOR USING INTERMITTENT FASTING TO ENHANCE MENTAL FOCUS

You can effectively improve your mental clarity and focus by engaging in intermittent fasting. However, do remember that the results don't just appear magically. Just like any skill, honing your focus during intermittent fasting requires a committed approach made up of several key strategies that play a crucial role, including the following:

- **Get enough sleep:** Sleep deprivation destroys your focus and is even more detrimental during fasting. Getting between seven and eight hours of sleep each night will be sufficient. Sleep deprivation impairs your cognitive function, reduces energy levels, and increases stress hormones, all of which hinder your ability to focus. Prioritize sleep as a foundational pillar for a sharp mind and a successful fasting experience.
- **Consume nourishing meals within your fasting periods:** While you may not be eating constantly during intermittent fasting, what you do eat during your feasting window matters immensely. Choose healthy, nutrient-dense options like whole foods, vegetables, healthy fats, lean proteins, and fruits. These options provide sustained energy and essential vitamins and minerals that support brain function. Avoid taking processed foods and sugary drinks, both of which can cause energy crashes and impair your focus. Remember, quality beats quantity, so make every bite count for optimal mental focus.
- **Avoid distractions:** Our modern world is filled with distractions, making it even harder to focus during intermittent fasting. Minimize distractions as much as possible. Create a dedicated workspace, silence your

phone notifications, and avoid multitasking. Utilize tools like noise-canceling headphones and time management apps to create a focused environment that enhances deeper concentration.

- **Stay active:** Regular exercise enhances your focus during intermittent fasting. Physical activity increases blood flow to the brain, delivers oxygen and nutrients, and stimulates the production of neurotransmitters like dopamine and endorphins. These neurotransmitters improve mood, cognitive function, and overall well-being. Whether it's a brief walk, yoga session, or mild strength-training exercise, incorporate movement into your fasting routine to keep your mind and body energized and focused.

- **Plan ahead:** Use planning your activities beforehand as a secret weapon for a smooth and focused fasting experience. Prepare your meals in advance and ensure that you have healthy options readily available when your eating window opens. Also, plan your work schedule and prioritize tasks that require high levels of focus during your peak energy periods. By anticipating your needs and having a plan in place, you minimize distractions and set yourself up for a successful fasting experience.

- **Break your fast with nutrient-dense foods:** Don't just break your fast with anything. Choose nutrient-dense foods that provide sustained energy and support cognitive function. Opt for foods that are rich in protein and complex carbohydrates, like eggs, avocado, berries, and oatmeal. Avoid sugary breakfast cereals or pastries, as these can cause blood sugar spikes and subsequent crashes, which can negatively impact your focus and energy levels throughout the day.

All these strategies are most effective when combined and tailored to suit your individual needs. Experiment to discover what works best for you, with prior medical consultations beforehand. With the right physical strategies and a personalized approach, you can use intermittent fasting to enhance your mental clarity and achieve focused success.

Mindfulness Practices

During intermittent fasting, managing energy fluctuations and staying mentally sharp can be challenging. However, incorporating mindfulness practices into your routine can be essential in enhancing your focus and helping you to walk your intermittent fasting journey with greater ease. Here are some mindfulness strategies to enhance your overall fasting experience:

- **Three-minute breathing space:** This simple yet powerful technique brings you into the present moment. Find a quiet spot, close your eyes, and simply observe your breath for three minutes. Notice the rise and fall of your chest, the temperature of the air, and the subtle sounds around you. Count each inhale and exhale without judgment while allowing any distractions to gently drift away. This practice calms your mind, reduces stress, and improves concentration.
- **Listening to mindfulness:** You can actively transform everyday activities into resources for enhancing mindfulness. For example, while washing dishes, fully immerse yourself in the experience. Listen attentively to the water movements, the clinking of plates, and the slimy feel of soap on your hands. Focus on the sensations and sounds without bias. This practice engages your senses,

quiets internal chatter, and enhances your presence in the moment, which naturally sharpens your focus.

- **Body scan:** This practice cultivates body awareness and promotes relaxation, which are both crucial elements for improved focus. Lie down comfortably and close your eyes. Begin by mentally scanning your toes while paying attention to any sensations like warmth, tingling, or tension. Slowly move your awareness upward, focusing on each body part impartially. This deepens your connection with your body and reduces mental noise. Overall, your awareness of the present is enhanced, leading to improved focus.

- **Four-seven-eight mindful breathing:** This calming technique is ideal for managing momentary overwhelm. Inhale deeply through your nose for four seconds, hold your breath comfortably for seven seconds, and then exhale slowly through your mouth for eight seconds. Repeat this cycle several times. This regulated breathing pattern stimulates the relaxation response, calms your nervous system, and improves cognitive function, thereby enhancing your ability to focus.

- **People-watching (mindfully):** Instead of mindlessly scrolling through your phone to observe people's activities, you can transform people-watching into a mindful activity. Observe people around you with curiosity. Notice their body language, facial expressions, and interactions. This practice engages your mind, sharpens your observational skills, and promotes present-moment awareness, thus ultimately enhancing your ability to focus and concentrate.

- **Group drawing:** This playful mindfulness exercise fosters a deep connection with those around you and increases present-moment awareness. Get together with a group of friends or colleagues and set a timer. Without looking at each other's drawings, select a theme or prompt, and then start drawing. Once the time is up, reveal your creations to each other and discuss the process. This activity encourages active listening, non-judgmental observation, and present-moment awareness, all of which contribute to enhanced focus.

Remember, consistency is key to reaping the benefits of these mindfulness practices. Start with shorter periods for each activity after finding what resonates with you, and then gradually integrate the practices into your daily routine. As you cultivate mindfulness, you'll not only experience enhanced focus during your fasting journey but also discover a deeper sense of calm and stay present.

DEALING WITH FATIGUE AND BRAIN FOG

Beginning intermittent fasting can be an exciting journey. However, you will likely face unwelcome experiences along the way. Fatigue and brain fog are the most common. While frustrating, understanding these symptoms and the explanations behind them will put you in a better position to manage them effectively. Some of the causes and explanations behind these symptoms are:

- **Adaptation period:** Your body is used to routine, and changing your eating patterns requires some adjustment. The initial days of fasting can involve your body switching its fuel sources. This may lead to temporary fatigue and sluggishness.
- **Low blood sugar:** Skipping meals can naturally dip your blood sugar levels, especially if you have pre-existing conditions like diabetes. This dip can manifest as fatigue, difficulty concentrating, or headaches. Stay hydrated and

keep focused on your body's signals to manage this. Break your fast immediately, if necessary.

- **Electrolyte imbalance:** Electrolytes like sodium, potassium, and magnesium play crucial roles in various bodily functions, including energy production and brain function. During fasting, electrolyte levels can fluctuate, thereby contributing to fatigue, muscle cramps, and brain fog. Replenishing electrolytes by taking natural sources like broth and coconut water and getting professional medical guidance will help you through.

- **Dehydration:** Dehydration is often masked as fatigue and brain fog. Even mild dehydration can impair your cognitive function and decrease your energy levels. To stay adequately hydrated and energized, ensure that you drink plenty of water, especially on fasting days.

- **Caloric deficit:** While weight loss is often a desired outcome of fasting, an excessive calorie deficit can be counterproductive. Restricting calories too much can lead to fatigue, decreased metabolism, and nutrient deficiencies. These symptoms all contribute to brain fog and sluggishness. Focus on balanced, nutrient-dense meals during your eating window to ensure that your body gets the fuel it needs for optimal function.

- **Metabolic transition:** As your body transitions from readily available glucose to ketone bodies for fuel during fasting, there can be a temporary dip in energy. This keto-adaptation period can last a few days to a few weeks, causing fatigue and brain fog. Be patient with your body if you experience this, and stay hydrated during this adjustment phase.

- **Stress and anxiety:** The stress of making dietary changes or the fear of the unknown can manifest as fatigue and brain fog. Prioritize stress management techniques like meditation, exercise, and adequate sleep to minimize their impact on your fasting experience.

Understanding the possible reasons for fatigue and brain fog and taking the necessary steps to address them allows you to endure the initial stages of intermittent fasting with greater ease and clarity.

PRACTICAL TIPS TO OVERCOME CHALLENGES

Here are practical tips to manage the common concerns arising during intermittent fasting:

- **Gradually adapt to fasting:** Start small. Instead of jumping into long fasts, start with brief durations like 12-hour windows and gradually lengthen them as your body adjusts. Also, don't push through discomfort. If you feel overly tired or lightheaded, break your fast, hydrate, eat balanced meals, and rest. If your symptoms continue or increase, call healthcare professionals.
- **Monitor caloric intake:** Track your calorific intake by using apps or a journal to track your calories during your eating window. Aim for a balanced, nutrient-dense approach that meets your individual needs. Also, focus on eating healthy foods. Choose calorie-rich, nutrient-dense foods like nuts, seeds, avocados, and fatty fish to ensure that your body gets essential nutrients.
- **Replenish electrolytes:** Include electrolyte-rich foods like coconut water, bone broth, leafy greens, and avocado in your diet. These are healthy natural sources of electrolytes. Consider consulting a healthcare professional for guidance on supplementing with potassium, magnesium, and

sodium, especially if you experience persistent cramps or
fatigue.

- **Include B vitamins:** Prioritize eating foods like eggs,
lentils, mushrooms, and leafy greens during your fast, as
these are rich in B vitamins, which are crucial for energy
metabolism and brain function. You may also need to
consult with a medical professional to determine if a B-
complex supplement might be beneficial, especially if
you're concerned about mineral deficiencies.
- **Maintain liver health:** Avoid harmful foods and
substances that damage your liver. Limit the intake of
alcohol and reduce the consumption of processed foods, as
these can burden your liver. Consume cruciferous
vegetables like broccoli and cauliflower, and take turmeric
and green tea, which are all known to support liver health.
- **Manage stomach acid levels:** Dilute a tablespoon of apple
cider vinegar in water before and during meals to aid
digestion and reduce heartburn. Also, avoid triggers to
stomach acid upset by refraining from foods like spicy
dishes, citrus fruits, and coffee, which can trigger
heartburn for some individuals. Ginger tea is a soothing
drink that can help to settle your stomach and reduce
discomfort.

The strategies for enhancing your mental focus and energy levels
during intermittent fasting were explained in this chapter. Fatigue
and brain fog are the main symptoms experienced during intermittent fasting that seem to work against the benefits of the practice. To avoid these, stay hydrated by drinking plenty of water, and
keep your energy levels replenished by eating foods like protein
and carbohydrates while avoiding processed foods. The chapter
also stressed the importance of keeping your mind clear and
achieving body calmness during intermittent fasting through

practices like mindful watching and regulated breathing. Once you attain a healthy mind and body during intermittent fasting, it becomes easier to incorporate exercise and physical activity to further enhance intermittent fasting's benefits. Let's dive into the next chapter to get detailed insight into this.

Make a Difference with Your Review: Unlock the Power of Generosity

"Thousands of candles can be lit from a single candle, and the candle's life will not be shortened. Happiness never decreases by being shared."

— BUDDHA

Leave a Quick Review!

Your feedback is invaluable and takes less than a minute. Help inspire others:

- Empower: Encourage better health and wellness.
- Motivate: Support others in their health journey.
- Educate: Share insights on balancing hormones and energy.

How to Leave a Review: Simply scan the QR code.

Join our community and let's promote a healthier, more energetic life together. Thank you for making a difference!

THE WEIGH TO WELLNESS

Roxanne constantly felt like a stranger in her own body. At 68, she could barely recognize the woman reflected in the mirror. She looked heavier and wearier than the energetic youth she remembered. Years of juggling work, family, and the convenience of quick, unhealthy meals had taken their toll. Her weight had gone up slowly, causing her clothes to feel much tighter. Roxanne knew things had to change. She had tried changing her diet and taking medication, but it all seemed in vain. She couldn't see any positive changes in her body. However, the desire to reclaim her health and energy still remained. Then, her friends encouraged her to try intermittent fasting. The concept of this dietary approach resonated with her practical nature, unlike restrictive diets.

The 16:8 method, with a daily fasting window of 16 hours and an eating period of only 8 hours, felt manageable to Roxanne. During her fasting windows, she gradually began feeling surprisingly clear-headed and energized. By the time her eating window opened, she felt genuinely hungry and was not mindlessly reaching for snacks. In no time, 10 pounds had vanished from her body, seemingly effortlessly, leaving behind a lighter and more energetic Roxanne. But the changes were more than just numerical. Her joints ached less, her sleep improved, and she started feeling more enthusiastic about going through her daily activities (Harlan, 2016). Just like Roxanne, you too can enjoy the numerous benefits of intermittent fasting. In this chapter, let me take you through some physical activities and exercises that are suitable for women over 50 that you can incorporate during your fasting windows. This chapter will focus on the letter **C** of the GRACE framework, which represents the word **C**ultivate, symbolizing how intermittent fasting nurtures weight management.

INTERMITTENT FASTING AND WEIGHT MANAGEMENT

Intermittent fasting has taken the health world by storm and is touted for its ability to aid weight management. But how exactly does it work? The key lies in its elaborate interlink with several critical factors that influence our weight, including:

Metabolic Impact

One of intermittent fasting's most compelling aspects is its metabolic impact. During a fast, your body gradually depletes its readily available glucose stores, thereby prompting a metabolic shift. Your body switches from its preferred glucose fuel source to using ketone bodies that are produced by the breaking down of stored fat by the liver. This metabolic switching is often lauded as the cornerstone of intermittent fasting's weight-loss benefits. Studies also suggest that intermittent fasting might also influence the metabolic rate itself. Some research indicates an increase in resting metabolic rate (RMR), which quantifies the calories that you utilize while resting (The University of Illinois, 2023). This translates to more calories burned throughout the day, even outside of your fasting periods. Additionally, enhanced insulin sensitivity, which allows your body to use glucose more efficiently, thereby preventing blood sugar spikes and subsequent cravings, can also be facilitated through intermittent fasting.

Fat Burning

While burning fat stores is crucial for weight loss, intermittent fasting's impact goes beyond simply getting rid of them. Fasting periods are thought to promote the release of hormones like glucagon, which signals the breakdown of fat for energy, according to research (Kang et al., 2022). Additionally, intermittent fasting is also thought to increase levels of norepinephrine, another hormone that stimulates fat-burning and lipolysis. Lipolysis is a process whereby your cells break down triglyceride fat molecules into fatty acids and glycerol. Furthermore, research suggests that fasting also influences autophagy, a cellular cleansing process where damaged cells are broken down and recycled, thereby improving metabolic efficiency, and reducing inflammation (Johns Hopkins Medicine, 2021). This coordination of hormonal changes and cellular processes creates an environment that is conducive to burning fat and reducing the overall body fat percentage.

Appetite Regulation

The relationship between intermittent fasting and appetite is complex and specific to each individual. While some individuals report reduced hunger and fewer cravings during fasting periods, others might experience initial discomfort. This variability partly stems from intermittent fasting's impact on hunger-regulating hormones. Fasting suppresses your levels of the hunger hormone, ghrelin, while increasing those of the satiety hormone, leptin (Kang et al., 2022).

There are variations in individual responses to intermittent fasting, depending on factors like your duration without eating, and personal dietary habits. Some individuals might initially experience increased hunger during fasting, which requires mindful strategies to manage. Nevertheless, research suggests that for many, intermittent fasting's appetite-regulating effects can contribute to reduced calorie intake and shedding extra pounds over time (Johns Hopkins Medicine, 2021).

RESEARCH THAT SUPPORTS INTERMITTENT FASTING'S ROLE IN WEIGHT MANAGEMENT

Intermittent fasting's weight loss potential has generated significant interest, with several studies supporting its effectiveness. A comprehensive analysis of 27 trials published in the Obesity Reviews Journal found that weight loss was observed in different individuals as a result of various intermittent fasting methods. The values of the lost pounds ranged from 0.8% to 13.0% of the initial body weight (Kang et al., 2022). Notably, this weight loss occurred regardless of whether participants changed their overall calorie intake, suggesting that the timing of eating might also play a crucial role.

The University of Illinois at Chicago published research findings that compared intermittent fasting to traditional calorie counting for weight loss. Their findings, published in the journal JAMA Internal Medicine, showed that both methods are equally effective, with participants losing between 3% and 8% of their body weight depending on the specific intermittent fasting approach that they used (The University of Illinois, 2023). The International Journal of Obesity published another study in which they investigated the

5:2 Plus dietary program, a particular intermittent fasting approach where participants go for five days on their normal diet and then restrict their food intake on two non-consecutive days to between 500 and 600 calories. This study found that an average of 8.5% body weight was lost by participants in just 12 weeks, along with reductions in waist circumference and other health markers (Kang et al., 2022).

STRATEGIES FOR WEIGHT MAINTENANCE THROUGH INTERMITTENT FASTING

Intermittent fasting offers a unique approach to weight management. It influences how your body utilizes energy by strategically cycling between your eating and fasting windows. Your body taps into stored fat reserves for fuel during fasting periods, resulting in weight reduction. Here are more strategies to help you manage your weight through intermittent fasting:

Meal Planning

Prioritize taking unprocessed varieties like vegetables, fruits, whole grains, and lean proteins. These foods pack powerful nutrients to keep you fuller for longer. Ensure that each meal incorporates protein, healthy fats, and complex carbohydrates for a balance of nutrition and sustained energy. Also, prepping your meals in advance helps you avoid unhealthy choices when hunger strikes during your eating window. In such cases, portion control becomes effortless, while healthier food choices are readily available. Remember to limit processed foods, sugary drinks, and refined carbohydrates. These options offer empty calories and can trigger cravings, thereby making weight maintenance difficult.

Mindful Eating

When you finally break your fast, remember to eat slowly and deliberately. Also, take careful note of your body's hunger signals. This prevents overeating and fosters a healthy relationship with food. Put away your phone and focus on your meal. Mindful eating allows you to appreciate flavors and textures, thus promoting better enjoyment and preventing mindless snacking. Opt for nutrient-rich meals that fuel your body and satisfy your taste buds. Limit sugary treats and processed foods that leave you craving more.

Managing Hunger During Your Fasting Window

Throughout the day, be sure to drink plenty of water to keep you feeling full and flush out toxins from your body. Drinking up to eight glasses or more of water is enough to keep you sufficiently hydrated. Also, remember to distract yourself by engaging in activities that you enjoy, exercising, or socializing to take your mind off food and make the fasting window easier to manage. If you are thinking of taking appetite suppressants during your fasting window to discourage yourself from eating, consult your doctor before doing so. Use these suppressants thoughtfully and only if medically necessary. You can also be sure to manage your hunger by enjoying black coffee in moderation. Black coffee can suppress your appetite and provide a small energy boost without breaking your fast. You may also use diluted apple cider vinegar to aid digestion and contribute to feeling fuller for longer. Lastly, sugar-free gum satisfies your urge to chew without adding unwanted calories. Choose minty flavors to help curb cravings.

EXERCISE SUGGESTIONS FOR WOMEN OVER 50

For a woman over 50, incorporating exercise into her fasting routine will play diverse roles in weight management. As her metabolism naturally slows down with age, maintaining her muscle mass becomes crucial. Exercise, therefore, acts as a counterweight that can preserve your muscle tissue, which in turn burns more calories even when you are at rest. Additionally, physical activity helps to regulate hormones like estrogen, which can fluctuate during peri- and post-menopause, thus influencing weight gain. Beyond weight management, exercise offers a multitude of benefits for you, including strengthening bones to combat osteoporosis, boosting energy levels, improving mood, and reducing your chances of chronic disease development.

Factors to Consider When Choosing Exercises

To ensure that you choose the right exercises that are compatible with what your body needs during intermittent fasting, consider the following factors:

- **Consult a healthcare provider:** Schedule a visit with a physician to discuss your fitness goals and any potential limitations. Your provider can guide you toward safe and effective exercise choices.
- **Engage in weight-bearing exercises:** Include weight-bearing exercises like walking, jogging, dancing, or lifting weights to build and maintain bone density and muscle mass.
- **Incorporate strength training:** Regular strength training with weights or body exercises builds stamina, improves balance, and boosts your metabolism.

- **Do aerobic activities:** Don't forget aerobic activities like brisk walking, swimming, or cycling for improved heart health, endurance, and mood.
- **Choose low-impact exercises:** Opt for low-impact exercises like swimming, water aerobics, or elliptical training to minimize stress on your joints.
- **Choose Tai Chi or Yoga:** These mind-body practices offer flexibility, balance, and stress reduction, promoting overall well-being.
- **Perform stretching exercises:** Regular stretching keeps your muscles flexible and helps to prevent injuries.
- **Start with moderate intensity:** Begin with moderate intensity and gradually increase duration and rigor over time to avoid strain.
- **Ensure exercise safety:** Consider how your body feels, both physically and emotionally, and take rest days whenever you feel the need to. Don't push yourself through pain. Use proper foam material to cushion your body and prevent injuries during exercise.
- **Gradually increase intensity:** Gradually increasing the intensity of your exercises challenges your body and keeps you motivated.
- **Select enjoyable activities:** Choose activities that you enjoy, whether it's dancing, Zumba, or hiking with friends. This makes exercise a pleasurable experience that you'll look forward to.
- **Participate in group classes:** Group exercise classes offer camaraderie, support, and motivation, which all make workouts more engaging.
- **Choose convenient exercises:** Choose exercises that fit comfortably into your schedule and lifestyle. Walk during your lunch break, try home workouts, or utilize gym facilities for this.

Suitable Exercises for Women Over 50

Here are some brief descriptions of a few strength-training exercises that are suitable for women over 50 like you:

- **Basic squat:** Stand with feet shoulder-width apart and toes slightly outward. Lower your body as if sitting back in a chair, keeping your back straight and your core engaged. Return to a standing position by pushing upward through your heels.
- **Modified push-up:** Start by getting into position on your knees, ensuring your hands are placed slightly wider than shoulder-width apart. Engage your core to maintain a straight line from your knees to your shoulders, then bend your elbows to lower your chest towards the ground before pushing back up to complete one repetition.
- **Incline push-up:** Place your hands on a sturdy surface like a bench or wall, further apart than shoulder-width. Extend your legs behind you, resting on the balls of your feet. The further back your feet are, the more challenging the push-up will be. Lower your chest toward the surface as you lean your body forward, keeping your back straight and your core engaged. Push back up to the starting position and repeat.
- **Seated row:** Sit with a resistance band looped around your feet or a cable machine. Pull the band or cable towards your chest, keeping your back straight and your core engaged. Release slowly to the starting position, then repeat.
- **Stationary lunge:** Space your feet hip-width apart while standing upright. Use one leg to step forward, then descend your body gently until you bend both knees at 90-

degree angles. Return to standing by pushing through your front heel. Use the other leg to repeat.

- **Walking lunges:** The procedure is the same as that of stationary lunges, but instead, step forward and alternate your legs continuously and walk instead of remaining stationary.
- **Dead bug:** Lie flat on your back with your arms extended straight up towards the ceiling, directly above your shoulders. Raise your legs, bending your knees at a 90-degree angle. Engage your core by pressing your lower back into the floor. Slowly lower your right arm and left leg toward the floor, straightening your leg and moving your arm backward over your head. Both limbs should move simultaneously and should only go as low as you can while keeping your lower back pressed to the floor. If your back starts to arch, you've gone too far.
- **Barbell bicep curl:** Stand with your feet spaced shoulder-width apart. Hold a barbell with an underhand grip at arm's length. Curl the weight towards your shoulder, keeping your upper arm close to your body. Lower yourself slowly back to the initial stance and repeat the cycle.
- **Single leg hamstring bridge:** Lie on your back with your knees bent and your feet flat on the ground. Lift your hips, while squeezing your glutes, and extend one leg upward toward the ceiling. Hold that position for a while, and then slowly lower your leg down to rest. Use the other leg to repeat the procedure.
- **Forearm plank:** Position yourself for a regular pushup, but rest on your forearms instead of your hands. Engage your core while keeping your body straight from head to toe. Maintain that stance for a while before repeating.

- **Bird dog:** Begin with your hands and knees on the floor, hands directly under your shoulders and knees under your hips. Simultaneously extend one arm forward and the opposite leg straight backward, while keeping your core engaged and your back flat. Maintain that position for a short moment before reverting to your initial point. Repeat with the other arm and leg.

The following are brief descriptions of some cardio exercises that are suitable for you:

- **Brisk walking:** Walk at a pace that gets your heart rate up and makes you slightly out of breath. Aim for at least 30 minutes most days of the week. You can walk outdoors, on a treadmill, or even indoors at a mall.
- **Swimming:** This is a low-impact, full-body workout that's gentle on your joints. You can do laps, swim freestyle, backstroke, breaststroke, or participate in water aerobics classes.
- **Dance exercise:** Choose a style that you enjoy, like Zumba, ballroom dancing, or hip-hop. Dance classes provide a fun and social way of increasing your heart rate and burning away some calories.
- **Indoor cycling:** Participate in spin cycling classes or cycle at your own pace. Adjust the resistance to match your fitness levels and enjoy a challenging cardio workout with low impact on your joints.
- **Water aerobics:** Join a group class or exercise on your own in a pool. This low-impact option offers a fun and refreshing way to improve your cardiovascular health and muscular strength.

- **Zumba:** This is a high-energy dance fitness class that incorporates Latin and international rhythms. Zumba is a fun way of burning calories and improving coordination.
- **Step aerobics:** Step aerobics is a high-energy cardio workout that involves stepping on and off a raised platform to the rhythm of music. Think of climbing stairs at a party pace! It tones your muscles, burns calories, and boosts coordination, all while adding a fun twist to traditional cardio.

There are exercises that loosen your muscles for easier movement and balance. Such exercises usually involve stretching and flexing your muscles. For safety reasons, I recommend that you stick to exercises that work well for your age, and these include the following:

- **Hip flexor stretch while kneeling:** Stand your foot firmly on the ground ahead of you while kneeling on one leg. Maintain a straight back and lean forward until your hip flexor muscles feel stretched. Hold for 30 seconds, and then repeat on your opposite side.
- **Calf stretch:** Stand facing a wall, about an arm's length away. Step one foot back, keeping it straight, with your heel firmly on the ground and your toes pointing straight ahead. The other foot should remain closer to the wall, with the knee slightly bent. Place your hands on the wall at shoulder height and lean forward, keeping your back straight. Press into the wall while keeping the heel of your back foot pressed firmly against the floor. Hold this position for 30 seconds before repeating the procedure.

- **Seated shoulder stretch:** Sit tall with your hands clasped behind your back. Gently push your palms down and lift your chest until you feel your shoulders and upper back being stretched. Hold for 30 seconds and release.
- **Seated hamstring stretch:** Sit on the floor with your legs extended straight in front of you. Keep your back straight and your toes pointing upwards. Bend one knee and place the sole of that foot against the inner thigh of your opposite leg, keeping the other leg straight. Slowly lean forward from your hips toward the extended leg, reaching towards your toes. Hold that position for 30 seconds and release before repeating on the opposite side.
- **Chest stretches:** Stand in a doorway with your forearms resting on either side of the frame. Lean forward, opening your chest and shoulders. Hold for 30 seconds and release before repeating.
- **Alternating arm reaches:** Reach one arm straight up overhead while standing with your feet spaced hip-width apart. Reach the other arm down toward your toes. Repeat on the other side after holding that position for a few seconds.
- **Seated spinal stretch:** Sit on the floor and extend your legs ahead of you. Lean forward, reaching for your toes or shins, while keeping your back straight. You can also interlace your fingers behind your back and gently push your palms down for a deeper stretch. Hold for 30 seconds and release yourself from the position before repeating.
- **Standing side reach:** Raise your arms overhead while standing with your feet hip-width apart. Lean slowly to one side, reaching your hand down toward your ankle or shin. Keep your other leg straight and avoid bending at the waist. Repeat on the other side after holding for about 30 seconds.

- **Hip and back stretch:** Bend both knees while lying on your back. Cross one ankle over the opposite thigh, just above the knee. Stretch your glutes by gently pulling the crossed leg toward your chest. Hold the position for 30 seconds and repeat on the other side.
- **Arm cross chest reach:** Lift your arms to shoulder height sideways while positioning your feet a considerable distance apart. Bend one elbow and bring your hand across your chest toward your opposite shoulder. Gently use your other hand to push your elbow deeper into the stretch. Hold the position for 30 seconds and repeat on the other side.

I also suggest the following balance exercises that are suitable for women over 50 like you:

- **Single-leg balance:** Stand on one leg while comfortably maintaining your balance for a considerable while. Repeat with the other leg. Aim to gradually increase the amount of time that you can hold each balance.
- **Tai Chi:** This ancient practice combines slow, gentle movements with deep breathing to improve balance, flexibility, and focus. Many community centers offer Tai Chi classes, so you are likely to find one near you.
- **Yoga:** Certain yoga poses, like mountain or tree poses, challenge your balance and core strength. Choose a beginner yoga class and focus on poses that specifically target balance.
- **Pilates:** This exercise method incorporates bodyweight movements and equipment to improve core strength, flexibility, and balance. Look for Pilates classes that are specifically designed for seniors.

- **Indoor walking workouts:** Use cones or markers to create an obstacle course indoors and walk over them. This exercise challenges your balance and coordination. You can also try heel-toe walking or side-shuffling exercises.

TIPS FOR STARTING AN EXERCISE ROUTINE

Before jumping into any workout, understand your body's needs and get your doctor's green light to continue. Find activities that you genuinely enjoy, whether it's a Zumba class, swimming laps, or brisk walks in nature. Start slow, aiming for shorter durations and lower intensity, gradually building up based on your comfort level. Also, remember to stay consistent with your physical routine. Your body easily adjusts to the routine over time. Set realistic goals and treat exercise like a date with yourself, so that it becomes a natural part of your healthy lifestyle. Also, remember that warming up with light stretches and low-impact movements prepares your body for the workout and helps to prevent injuries. Here are some handy tips that you can use to start up your exercise routine:

- **The high knees warm-up routine:** Stand upright, with your hands resting by your belly button. Now, march in place, bringing each knee up powerfully to meet your palm. Keep it going for between 20 and 30 marches. For an extra twist, add ankle circles while you pump your knees. This exercise is quite simple yet very effective, as it gets your legs warm, loose, and ready for your workout while improving your overall coordination.
- **The shoulder roll exercise:** This warmup exercise removes stiffness and gets your shoulders ready to move freely. Space your feet shoulder-width apart while standing upright. Allow your arms to hang relaxed by your

sides. Now, imagine that you're trying to reach your ears with your shoulders, shrugging them up high, and then rolling them back and down like circles drawn on your back. Keep those circles going, aiming for between eight and ten in each direction.

- **Bent-arm shoulder rotation exercise:** This warmup exercise unleashes your shoulder mobility. Widen your arms on either side, keeping them slightly lower than shoulder height, while you are standing upright. Bend your elbows, forming 90-degree angles, and imagine you're drawing tiny circles with your forearms. Rotate your elbows in small forward circles, up to 15 times, and then reverse the direction for another set.
- **Arm swing exercise:** Plant your feet firmly on the ground. Gently rotate your upper body to the right, letting your arms swing freely in the opposite direction. Feel the movement flowing through your arms, and shoulders and giving your spine a gentle twist. Swing back and forth, repeating the rotations several times on each side.
- **Cardio warm-up exercises:** Lace up your shoes and take a brisk walk around the block. This warmup exercise isn't a race, but the goal is to gently elevate your heart rate and blood flow. This prepares your body for more intense activity. Remember to keep the pace moderate. Use the talk test to determine if your pace is moderate. If you can comfortably speak two sentences in a row without running out of breath, then you are doing just fine. You should feel warm, but not breathless.

To optimize your health through intermittent fasting, it's essential to strategically prepare for exercise as well. Incorporating mobility exercises, such as stretching before and after workouts, is crucial for maintaining muscle health and flexibility. Additionally, techniques like foam rolling, massage, or utilizing heat and cold therapies can significantly enhance your workout experience and facilitate muscle recovery. Embracing these practices ensures your body is primed for peak performance and swift recovery, aligning with your intermittent fasting goals for holistic well-being.

This chapter has guided you through integrating physical exercise and activities to complement your intermittent fasting journey, aimed at healthy weight management. It highlighted scientific evidence that underscores the benefits of fasting on metabolism, fat burning, and appetite regulation, reinforcing the effectiveness of these practices. To augment your weight management efforts, strategies such as mindful eating, meal planning, and managing hunger during fasting periods were discussed. Additionally, we recommended physical activities specifically chosen to synergize with intermittent fasting, ensuring your body remains in top condition. These exercises will produce excellent results when you incorporate a healthy diet into your fasting routine. Moving forward into the next chapter, we will delve into mindful eating, providing a comprehensive guide to nourishing your body optimally during fasting.

NOURISHING YOUR FASTING BODY

Ava Safir, a registered dietitian, was intrigued by the buzz surrounding the 16:8 intermittent fasting approach. However, the thought of working out while in a fasted state initially worried her. She wondered if she could maintain her energy throughout the exercise routines without negatively impacting her performance. Taking her chances, she decided to start slow, opting for walks and gentle yoga during her fasting window. To her surprise, she felt focused and energized. Soon, she was incorporating strength training, proving to herself that preconceived notions could be challenged. What truly surprised Ava, however, was the change in her relationship with food. Breaking her fast with wholesome, vibrant breakfasts became a daily joy. She embraced intuitive eating by tuning into her body's demands to eat, rather than relying on rigid meal plans.

The only downside to this was not being able to share breakfast with her family, as their feeding schedules fell within her fasting window. However, Ava remained positive and began connecting with her family outside of mealtimes by cherishing quality conversations and shared activities. Her ultimate goal through intermittent fasting wasn't actually weight loss, but embracing a healthier lifestyle. Ultimately, the experiment with the 16:8 intermittent fasting approach solidified her belief in using personalized approaches to attain healthy living. Intermittent fasting might have worked for her, but the key was listening to her body and adapting the approach to fit her unique needs and preferences. This chapter details the letter **E** of the GRACE framework's acronym, which represents the Enrichment section. Let's share more insight on this as you keep reading through.

THE IMPORTANCE OF NUTRITION IN INTERMITTENT FASTING

Intermittent fasting's health benefits range from weight management to improved cognitive function, making it an enticing dietary option. However, maximizing these benefits relies heavily on proper nutrition during your eating window. Here's how:

- **Weight management:** Intermittent fasting restricts calorie intake, thereby leading to weight loss. However, taking nutrient-dense food options during your eating window ensures that you're adequately fueled and helps to avoid rebound food binging. An endocrinology review found intermittent fasting's effectiveness for weight loss to be similar to that of continuous calorie restriction. Studies using healthy dietary patterns during eating windows also showed better weight loss maintenance compared to those with less emphasis on nutrient quality (Johns Hopkins Medicine, 2021).

- **Enhanced control of blood sugar:** Insulin sensitivity and reduced blood sugar levels can be achieved through intermittent fasting. However, choosing low-glycemic index (GI) carbohydrates further stabilizes blood sugar and reduces cravings. The JAMA Internal Medicine study in 2017 found that individuals with type 2 diabetes achieved enhanced insulin sensitivity and long-term blood sugar control through intermittent fasting (Ackerman, 2019). Adding low-GI carbohydrates to intermittent fasting diets further improved these outcomes.

- **Better heart health:** Intermittent fasting can help to reduce inflammation, regulate cholesterol levels, and lower your blood pressure. However, emphasizing heart-healthy fats like omega-3s and monounsaturated options further optimizes these benefits. Research has found that a Mediterranean diet that is rich in healthy fats, when incorporated into intermittent fasting, significantly reduces LDL, known as bad cholesterol, and improves HDL, also termed good cholesterol (Ackerman, 2019).

- **Reduced inflammation:** Intermittent fasting can decrease pro-inflammatory markers in your body. However, consuming anti-inflammatory foods like fruits, vegetables, and spices further minimizes inflammation. Studies in cell metabolism found that inflammatory markers in individuals with obesity were significantly reduced by practicing intermittent fasting (Johns Hopkins Medicine, 2021). Research that investigated healthy dietary patterns during intermittent fasting showed even greater reductions in inflammation.

- **Increased energy levels:** Intermittent fasting can induce ketosis, whereby your body utilizes fat for energy, thereby increasing your energy levels. However, consuming adequate protein ensures sustained energy and prevents muscle breakdown. Research has shown that intermittent fasting increases fat burning and promotes cellular adaptations that enhance energy production. Studies emphasizing sufficient protein intake during intermittent fasting also show better energy level maintenance and improved exercise performance (Johns Hopkins Medicine, 2021).

- **Stronger bones and muscles:** Intermittent fasting can stimulate the production of growth hormone, which is beneficial for bone and muscle health. However, consuming adequate calcium and vitamin D ensures even better bone health, and consuming a protein-rich diet helps to maintain muscle mass. A study in cell reports found that intermittent fasting increased growth hormone levels, thus making it beneficial for bone density. Studies combining intermittent fasting with adequate protein intake showed no muscle loss and even some gain in certain individuals (Ackerman, 2019).

- **Reduced chronic disease risk:** Intermittent fasting is thought to improve various metabolic markers that are linked to chronic conditions like heart disease and diabetes. However, consuming a balanced diet rich in fruits, vegetables, whole grains, and lean protein provides essential nutrients to combat these diseases. Observational studies also suggest intermittent fasting's possible merits in reducing the risk of certain chronic diseases. However, more research is still needed to confirm these findings (Johns Hopkins Medicine, 2021).

- **Healthy aging:** Intermittent fasting promotes cellular repair and longevity pathways. Additionally, these benefits can be enhanced by consuming antioxidants found in fruits, vegetables, and certain spices. Animal studies showed that intermittent fasting may extend lifespan and improve certain markers of aging (Johns Hopkins Medicine, 2021).

LISTENING TO YOUR BODY'S NEEDS

Mindful eating is the practice of paying close attention to the sensations and emotions surrounding your food choices. It stands as a powerful complement to your intermittent fasting experience. While intermittent fasting restricts when you eat, mindful eating focuses on how you eat, thus offering a holistic approach to nourishing your body and mind. The coordination between these two practices lies in their shared emphasis on self-awareness. Intermittent fasting fosters awareness of your body's hunger and satiety cues, thereby guiding your eating window. Mindful eating takes this a step further by tuning you into the internal experience of eating itself. You observe your emotions, thoughts, and physical sensations throughout the process, consequently creating a deeper understanding of your relationship with food. This enhanced self-awareness translates into several benefits for your fasting journey, including:

- **Healthier eating habits:** Mindful eating encourages you to enjoy your food, chew thoroughly, and appreciate the meal quality over the amount. This naturally leads to more mindful food choices during your eating window, thus promoting the selection of nutrient-dense, whole foods over processed options. You're less likely to mindlessly overeat or succumb to cravings as you become more attuned to your body's true needs.
- **Improved self-discipline:** The practice of observing your thoughts and emotions around food, without judgment, strengthens your self-discipline. As you become aware of your triggers for unhealthy choices, you're empowered to

make conscious decisions aligned with your goals. This self-discipline applies not just to your eating window but also to maintaining your fasting period without succumbing to temptations.

- **Sustainable weight management:** Mindful eating promotes a non-restrictive mindset toward food by shifting the focus from weight loss to mindful nourishment. This aligns perfectly with the long-term sustainability goals of intermittent fasting and prevents the back-and-forth patterns that are often associated with restrictive diets.

- **Increased enjoyment:** When you truly pay attention to your food, you develop a deeper appreciation for its taste, texture, and aroma. This mindful enjoyment enhances the pleasure of eating and transforms meals into mindful experiences rather than just feeding periods. This increased enjoyment can further support adherence to your intermittent fasting protocol.

- **Emotional regulation:** Mindful eating helps you identify emotional triggers for unhealthy eating patterns, like stress-induced snacking. By acknowledging these emotions without judgment, you can develop healthier coping mechanisms, thus preventing emotional eating during your fasting window or making unhealthy choices within your eating period.

Mindful eating and intermittent fasting complement each other beautifully. If you can cultivate self-awareness and foster healthier habits, mindful eating can maximize the full possibilities of intermittent fasting. It can transform the practice from a dietary approach into a mindful lifestyle that nourishes both your body and mind. Its true benefits lie not just in what you eat or when, but also in how you approach the entire nourishment experience.

Strategies for Practicing Mindful Eating

Mindful eating isn't just about controlling what you eat; it's about how you experience food. Here's a breakdown of key strategies for practicing mindful eating, with some practical tips to incorporate them into your life:

- **Make eating an exclusive event:** Treat meals as dedicated experiences, not rushed activities. Sit down at a table, avoid TV or electronic devices, and focus solely on the act of eating. Set designated mealtimes, clear distractions from your table, and engage in conversation with those you're eating with.
- **Eat slowly:** Savor each bite, chewing thoroughly, and allow your body time to register fullness signals. Put down your utensil after each bite, focus on the texture and flavors, and avoid multitasking while eating.
- **Turn off distractions:** Eliminate distractions like TV, music, or work, that compete with your attention to your eating experience. Silence your phone notifications, create a calming atmosphere during meals, and avoid rushing from one activity to another.
- **Take heed of your body's hunger cues:** Be attentive to your hunger pangs and satiety signals during intermittent fasting. Eat until you're comfortably full, not stuffed. Check in with your body before, during, and after meals. Ask yourself if you're truly hungry or just emotionally driven to eat. Stop when you're comfortably full, not overwhelmed.
- **Check your stress level:** Identify emotional triggers for unhealthy eating and develop healthier coping mechanisms to manage stress. Practice mindfulness exercises like deep breathing or meditation to manage

stress. Seek healthy outlets for emotional release, like exercise or spending time in nature.

- **Appreciate your food:** Take time to acknowledge the effort and resources involved in bringing food to your plate. Cultivate gratitude for the nourishment it provides. Before eating, reflect on the journey of your food, from farm to table. Express gratitude for the farmers, producers, and others who are involved in its creation.
- **Notice the details:** Engage all your senses in the eating experience. Pay attention to the flavors, textures, aromas, and colors of your food. Take a moment to visually appreciate your food before eating. Close your eyes and smell the aromas. Savor the different textures and flavors in each bite.
- **Cultivate a mindful kitchen:** Create an environment that encourages healthy eating habits. Stock your kitchen with nutritious options and remove tempting triggers. Organize your pantry and fridge to prioritize healthy options. Remove sugary drinks and processed foods from sight. Keep fresh fruits and vegetables readily available.
- **Practice non-judgment:** Accept your eating habits without judgment. Recognize cravings and setbacks as learning opportunities. Be kind to yourself. Acknowledge that mindful eating is a journey, not a destination. Forgive yourself for occasional slip-ups and focus on progress, not perfection.

Mindful eating is a practice, not a perfectionist pursuit. Incorporating these strategies into your daily life allows you to cultivate a more conscious and enjoyable relationship with food.

Listening to Your Body's Needs During Intermittent Fasting

Intermittent fasting hinges on understanding your body's cues and respecting its needs. Here's a deeper insight into how to truly listen to your body during intermittent fasting:

- **Recognize hunger cues:** Ditch looking at the clock to determine when to break your fast, and start listening to your stomach. True hunger often arrives as a gradual gnawing or rumbling sensation in your stomach, which is sometimes accompanied by mild fatigue or a subtle desire to eat. Ignoring these internal signals can lead to overeating much later.
- **Honor your fullness cues:** Just like recognizing hunger, pay close attention to when you feel comfortably full. This is not about feeling stuffed but rather about a sense of satisfaction and satiety. Stopping at this point allows your body to process the food efficiently and prevents unnecessary calorie intake.
- **Differentiate between hunger and other cues:** Don't let your brain trick you. Sometimes, thirst, boredom, stress, or even your eating habits can masquerade as hunger. Regularly ask yourself when was the last time that you drank water and whether or not you are feeling restless or emotionally charged. Your responses to this personal inquisition will determine whether the urge to break your fast is just a craving or a true hunger cue. Dehydration, boredom, and stress often have quick, healthy fixes that will allow you to continue your fast without any issues, rather than taking food.
- **Avoid emotional eating:** We all have emotional connections to food. However, during intermittent fasting, it's crucial to separate emotional needs from true hunger.

If you find yourself reaching for food due to stress, sadness, or frustration, try alternative coping mechanisms like meditation, exercise, or journaling.

- **Listen to your energy levels:** Feeling sluggish or foggy doesn't always mean that you're hungry. Carefully consider if your energy dip could be related to sleep deprivation, a lack of physical activity, or dehydration. If low energy persists over time, consult a healthcare professional for a medical assessment.
- **Monitor your mood:** Food can impact your mood. Nonetheless, be mindful if you're using it as a quick fix for emotional swings. Pay attention to how different foods affect your mood and seek healthier ways to manage emotions, like spending time in nature or connecting with loved ones.
- **Get professional healthcare guidance:** Seeking professional healthcare guidance prior to commencing fasting is crucial if you're unsure about interpreting your body's cues. This is especially the case if you have any underlying medical issues. They can help you tailor your intermittent fasting approach to your unique needs and ensure that you're listening to your body safely and effectively.

Paying attention to your body is a skill that takes practice and patience. Experiment with different strategies, track your experiences in a journal and be kind to yourself as you learn and adapt. The key is to move beyond rigid schedules and reconnect with your body's innate wisdom, thereby making intermittent fasting a truly personalized and sustainable journey.

WHAT TO EAT DURING EATING WINDOWS FOR OPTIMAL HEALTH

While intermittent fasting restricts your eating window, what you choose to fuel your body during that time significantly impacts your overall health and weight management. Here's a breakdown of some key strategies for making the most of your eating window:

- **Follow a balanced diet:** Opt for a diet that is rich in diverse, nutrient-dense whole foods, like the Mediterranean diet. This approach emphasizes leafy greens and vegetables that are abundant in fiber, vitamins, and minerals. These foods add volume and essential nutrients to your meals. Healthy fats like omega-3 fatty acids that are found in fish, nuts, and avocados, and which promote heart health and satiety are also recommended. Incorporating lean protein sources like fish, beans, lentils, and poultry will provide essential amino acids for muscle building and repair. Brown rice, quinoa, and whole-wheat bread are good options for sustained energy and fiber intake.

- **Choose nutrient-dense foods:** Prioritize foods that are packed with fiber, minerals, and vitamins over empty calories. Focus on beans and lentils to provide protein, fiber, and essential minerals like iron and magnesium. Eggs are another affordable and readily available source of protein, healthy fats, and choline, which are important for brain health. Fish is also a nutrient-dense option that contains omega-3 fatty acids in abundance. These are good for heart and brain health and are an excellent source of lean protein. Nuts and avocados are other nutrient-dense food options that provide healthy fats, fiber, and various vitamins and minerals for promoting satiety and overall well-being.

- **Water and electrolyte drinks:** Stay sufficiently hydrated during your intermittent fast. Water is essential for overall health and can help curb cravings during your fasting window. For essential electrolytes that are lost through sweat, especially during longer fasts, consider taking unsweetened herbal teas or electrolyte-supplemented water.
- **Avoid overeating:** Although you have a limited eating window during intermittent fasting, mindful eating still applies. Avoid mindlessly overeating, especially with unhealthy options. Attend to your body's hunger and satiety cues, and remember to stop eating once you feel satisfied, and not stuffed. Also, decide what you will eat beforehand to avoid impulsive choices. Lastly, focus on the food's nutritional value over volume. Nutrient-dense foods provide more satisfaction with much smaller portions compared to unhealthy options.
- **Limit processed foods:** Minimize processed foods, sugary drinks, and unhealthy fats. These offer little nutritional value, can spike blood sugar levels, and also lead to cravings, which can negatively affect your fast.
- **Consider protein and fiber:** If you are taking calories during your fast, prioritize taking protein- and fiber-rich foods. These can promote satiety, regulate blood sugar, and prevent muscle loss.

This chapter has given you a heads-up on tips for keeping your body nourished during your intermittent fast. The key is to include wholesome foods in your meals and keep your hydration optimized by taking lots of water or healthy liquids like coffee. However, remember to avoid overeating when you break your fast, as this can act to reverse the benefits of fasting. The chapter also enlightened you on strategies for mindful eating, like eating slowly, appreciating your food, and being in an environment that encourages healthy eating. With these tips in mind, you are all set to prepare heart-healthy recipes during your intermittent fast to make the experience more enjoyable. Join me in the next chapter as I put together some delicious recipes to add a spark to your fasting experience!

HEART-HEALTHY RECIPES FOR INTERMITTENT FASTING

Kate's initial attempt at intermittent fasting was irregular. Food cravings continuously disturbed her resolve, and her weight just wouldn't change. Determined to improve, she began trying combinations of different intermittent fasting recipes to discover new flavors that defied "diet food" stereotypes. Spicy lentil stews replaced bland salads, breakfast burritos filled with fluffy eggs and veggies offered protein-packed mornings, and her beloved peanut butter smoothies were transformed with protein powder and spinach, becoming a post-workout delight. As the weeks turned into months, Kate noticed a shift. Not just in the numbers on the scale, which showed a glorious 6-pound drop, but in her energy levels and overall well-being. Now, ready to build on Kate's journey and inspire others, I have embarked on the adventure of creating a section in this book that is filled with mouth-watering recipes specifically designed for intermittent fasting. This chapter will take you on a journey to unlock the secrets to healthy and satisfying meals that will fund your energy reservoirs during your fasting periods. Healthy eating will also help you break through plateaus. This chapter touches on the Enrich segment of the GRACE framework and proves to you that the words delicious and nutritious can actually go hand-in-hand on your intermittent fasting journey.

NOURISHING AND DELICIOUS SAVORY RECIPES

Are you craving flavor without sacrificing your health? Well, look no further. Explore these delightful savory recipes, packed with wholesome ingredients and bursting with taste. From protein-rich options to vibrant vegetarian delights, these dishes will satisfy your appetite and nourish your body. Let's get cooking!

Heart-Healthy Recipes

Let's break the boring meal routine with these interesting dishes!

Chile-Lime Tilapia with Corn Sauté
(BHG Test Kitchen, 2018)

Enjoy a zesty fiesta on a plate!

Ingredients

- 2 tilapia fillets
- 1 tablespoon olive oil
- 1 teaspoon chili powder
- 1/2 teaspoon cumin
- 1/4 teaspoon garlic powder
- pinch of salt and pepper
- 1/2 cup fresh corn kernels
- 1/4 cup each of red bell pepper, green bell pepper, red onion, fresh cilantro, all diced and chopped
- 1 tablespoon lime juice

Instructions

1. Combine olive oil, garlic powder, cumin, chili powder, salt, and pepper in a bowl. Rub the mixture onto both sides of the tilapia fillets.
2. Use medium heat on a large skillet. Add tilapia and cook for four to five minutes on each side.
3. While the Tilapia cooks, heat another tablespoon of olive oil in a separate pan. Add corn, bell peppers, and onion. Cook for about five to seven minutes, until these ingredients are softened. Stir in cilantro and lime juice.
4. Serve Tilapia over the corn sauté and enjoy!

Nutritional information: 350 calories, 25 g carbohydrates, 35 g protein, and 15 g fat per serving.

Seared Salmon with Pistachio Gremolata (BHG Test Kitchen, 2017)

Salmon bliss with a nutty crunch!

Ingredients

- 2 salmon fillets
- 1 tablespoon each of olive oil, lemon zest, and chopped fresh parsley
- 1/4 cup shelled pistachios, roughly chopped
- 1/4 teaspoon garlic powder
- pinch of salt and pepper

Instructions

1. Over medium-high heat, preheat a skillet. Coat the inside of the skillet with olive oil.
2. Pat the salmon dry and add salt and pepper seasoning. Place skin-side down in the hot skillet and cook for 4 to 5 minutes, until crispy. Flip and cook for another 2 to 3 minutes, or until desired doneness.
3. Meanwhile, combine chopped pistachios, lemon zest, parsley, garlic powder, and a pinch of salt in a small bowl.
4. Top the cooked Salmon with the pistachio gremolata and serve immediately.

Nutritional Information: 400 calories, 5 g carbohydrates, 30 g protein, and 30 g fat per serving.

Balsamic Chicken and Vegetables
(BHG Test Kitchen, 2011)

Enjoy this oven-roasted, tangy delight!

Ingredients

- 2 chicken breasts, skinless and boneless
- 1 tablespoon each of olive oil, honey
- 1/2 teaspoon oregano, dried
- 1/4 teaspoon garlic powder
- pinch of salt and pepper
- 1 each of red bell pepper, yellow bell pepper, and onion, sliced
- 1/4 cup balsamic vinegar
- 1/4 cup fresh parsley, chopped

Instructions

1. Set the oven temperature to 400 °F.
2. Add olive oil, garlic powder, salt, oregano, and pepper to a small bowl and mix well. Rub the mixture on both sides of the chicken breasts.
3. Arrange the chicken and vegetables on a baking sheet in a single layer.
4. Whisk together balsamic vinegar and honey in a separate bowl. Drizzle evenly over the chicken and vegetables.
5. Roast for about 23 minutes. The vegetables should be tender by then.
6. Use fresh parsley to garnish. Serve.

Nutritional Information: 450 calories, 25 g carbohydrates, 40 g proteins, and 20 g fat per serving.

Oven-Roasted Salmon with Charred Lemon Vinaigrette (Woman Day's Kitchen, 2019)

Lemony goodness with a smoky twist!

Ingredients

- 2 salmon fillets
- 1 tablespoon olive oil
- 1/4 cup water
- pinch of pepper and salt
- 1 tablespoon each Dijon mustard, honey
- 1/2 lemon, sliced
- 1/4 teaspoon thyme, dried

Instructions

1. Preheat the oven to 400 °F. Broil the lemon halves, cut side up, for 5 minutes until charred. Transfer to a plate and set aside.
2. On a rimmed baking sheet, toss fennel and onions with 1 tablespoon olive oil, 1/8 teaspoon salt, and 1/8 teaspoon pepper. Arrange vegetables around the edges of the sheet.
3. Season the salmon with the remaining 1/8 teaspoon salt and pepper. Place skin-side-down in the center of the sheet.
4. Roast for about 20 minutes until a fork can easily flake the salmon.
5. While the salmon roasts, juice the charred lemons into a small bowl. Whisk in mustard, water, and the remaining tablespoon of olive oil. Add salt and pepper seasoning to taste.
6. Take the salmon out of the oven and leave it for five minutes. Flake salmon with a fork.
7. Toss arugula with vinaigrette and arrange on plates. Top with roasted vegetables and flaked salmon. Drizzle with any remaining vinaigrette.

Nutritional information: 430 calories, 17 g carbohydrates, 42 g protein, 4 g fat, and 4 g fiber per serving.

Chicken Kebabs
(Sheff, 2018)

Enjoy a skewered flavor sizzle on your tongue!

Ingredients

- 1 chicken breasts, boneless, cubed, skinless
- 1/2 of each red bell pepper, green bell pepper, cubed
- 1 of each zucchini, red onion, cubed
- 1 tablespoon olive oil
- 1 teaspoon paprika
- 1/2 teaspoon garlic powder
- 1/4 teaspoon each of salt, black pepper

Instructions

1. Preheat the oven to 400 °F.
2. In a bowl, toss chicken with olive oil, spices, and salt/pepper.
3. Thread chicken and vegetables onto skewers, alternating colors and textures.
4. Place skewers on a clean baking sheet. Bake for no more than 25 minutes.

Nutritional information: 300 calories, 15 g carbohydrates, 35 g proteins, 10 g fat, and 2 g fiber.

Roasted Asparagus, Fish, and Bay Leaves
(BHG Test Kitchen, 2017)

A Mediterranean fusion!

Ingredients

- 1 pound asparagus spears, trimmed
- 1 pound white fish fillets, cod or haddock
- 4 fresh bay leaves
- 2 tablespoons olive oil
- 1/2 lemon, juiced
- 1/2 teaspoon each of garlic powder, salt, black pepper

Instructions

1. Preheat the oven temperature to 400 °F.
2. Toss in asparagus with salt, pepper, garlic powder, and 1 tablespoon olive oil.
3. Arrange asparagus on a baking sheet. Place the fish fillets on top and top each with a bay leaf.
4. Drizzle the remaining lemon juice and olive oil over the fish.
5. Bake for up to 20 minutes, until the fish is cooked through and flakes easily.

Nutritional information: 350 calories, 5 g carbohydrates, 40 g protein, 15 g fat, and 2 g fiber per serving.

Skillet Lasagna
(BHG Kitchen, 2016)

Where taste meets convenience!

Ingredients

- 1 tablespoon olive oil
- 1/2 onion, diced
- 1/4 cup Parmesan cheese, grated
- 1/4 cup baby spinach
- 14 ounces tomatoes, crushed
- 2 cloves garlic, minced
- 1 pound ground turkey or lean beef
- 1/2 cup low-fat ricotta cheese
- 8 ounces whole-wheat lasagna noodles, cooked
- salt and pepper, to taste

Instructions

1. Put olive oil in a skillet and warm it over medium heat. Add the onion and cook until softened.
2. Add garlic before further cooking for another minute.
3. Crumble in the ground meat and cook until browned. Drain any excess fat.
4. Stir in crushed tomatoes, ricotta cheese, Parmesan cheese, and salt and pepper. Simmer for 10 minutes.
5. Add cooked lasagna noodles, breaking them as needed to fit the skillet.
6. Add spinach, stir, and simmer for not more than seven minutes.

Nutritional information: 400 calories, 30 g carbohydrates, 35 g protein, 15 g fat, and 4 g fiber per serving.

Hot Honey-Glazed Salmon with Radishes
(Hurwitz and Berry, 2022)

A sweet and spicy treat!

Ingredients

- 1 pound salmon fillets, with skin-on
- 1/2 bunch radishes, trimmed, halved radishes
- 1 tablespoon olive oil
- 1/2 teaspoon salt
- 1/2 teaspoon black pepper
- 2 tablespoons honey
- sriracha sauce, adjusted to the desired spice level

Instructions

1. Beforehand, heat the oven to 400 °F. Toss radishes with oil, salt, and pepper. Spread it on a baking sheet.
2. Place the salmon fillets, skin-side down, on a separate baking sheet. In a small bowl, mix honey and Sriracha. Brush half the mixture over the salmon.
3. Roast both sheets for approximately 20 minutes. Brush the salmon with the remaining glaze before serving.

Nutritional information per serving: 450 calories, 15 g carbohydrates, 40 g protein, 25 g fat, and 2 g fiber.

Salmon with Lemon and Herbs
(Perri, 2020)

Enjoy simple elegance!

Ingredients

- 1 pound salmon fillets, skin-on
- 1 lemon, sliced thin
- 1 tablespoon fresh dill, chopped
- 1 teaspoon fresh parsley, chopped
- 1/2 teaspoon garlic powder
- 1/4 teaspoon salt, black pepper

Instructions

1. Preheat your oven to a temperature of 400 °F. Arrange lemon slices on a baking sheet. Place the salmon fillets, skin-side down, on top.
2. Sprinkle dill, parsley, garlic powder, salt, and pepper over the salmon.
3. Bake for 20 minutes to ensure that the salmon is cooked through.

Nutritional information: 400 calories, 5 g carbohydrates, 45 g protein, 20 g fat, 1 g fiber.

Heart-Healthy Recipes That Aid Weight Loss

Are you craving delicious meals that support your heart health and weight-management goals? Well, look no further! Explore these flavorful recipes featuring ingredients that are rich in nutrients and fiber, all designed to keep you satisfied and on track during your intermittent fast.

Salmon-Stuffed Avocados
(Gellman, 2023)

Where creamy ingredients meet!

Ingredients

- 2 halved and pitted ripe avocados
- 1/4 teaspoon Dijon mustard
- 10 ounces canned salmon, flaked
- 1 tablespoon each, chopped fresh dill, lemon juice
- 1/4 cup red onion, diced
- salt and pepper, to taste

Instructions

1. Scoop out some flesh from each avocado half, leaving a border. Mash avocado flesh with lemon juice, mustard, salt, and pepper.
2. Combine flaked salmon, red onion, and dill. Gently fold in the mashed avocado mixture.
3. Stuff avocado halves with the salmon mixture and enjoy!

Nutritional information: 450 calories, 10 g carbohydrates, 30 g protein, 30 g fat, and 5 g fiber.

Kale and White Bean Potpie with Chive Biscuits
(Killeen, 2023b)

Savory surprise for your tastebuds!

Ingredients

- 1 onion, diced
- 2 cloves garlic, minced
- 4 cups kale, chopped
- 1 can each of diced tomatoes
- 1 tablespoon olive oil
- 1 can rinsed white beans, drained
- 1/2 cup vegetable broth
- 1 teaspoon thyme, dried
- salt and pepper to taste
- 1 cup self-rising flour
- 1/4 cup each of cold cubed unsalted butter, chopped fresh chives
- 1/2 cup milk

Instructions

1. Preheat the oven to 400 °F. Prepare biscuit dough (combine flour, butter, chives, and milk until crumbly, then add milk until a soft dough forms).
2. Add oil to a pot and heat over medium heat. Sauté the onion until softened. Add garlic and cook for another minute.
3. Stir in kale, tomatoes, white beans, broth, thyme, salt, and pepper. Simmer for 10 minutes.
4. Pour the potpie filling into a baking dish.

5. Add biscuit dough to the filling before baking for about 25 minutes. The biscuits will become golden brown by then.

Nutritional information: 400 calories, 40 g carbohydrate, 20 g protein, 15 g fat, and 10 g fiber per serving.

Summer Vegetable Gnocchi Salad
(O'Brien, 2023)

Light and vibrant delicacy!

Ingredients

- 1 package whole-wheat gnocchi, cooked according to package instructions
- 1 cup cherry tomatoes, halved
- 1/2 diced cucumber
- 1 tablespoon lemon juice
- 1/4 cup fresh basil, chopped
- 1/2 cup feta cheese, crumbled
- 2 tablespoons olive oil
- salt and pepper to taste

Instructions

1. Cook gnocchi according to package directions. Cool slightly.
2. Combine gnocchi, tomatoes, cucumber, feta cheese, and basil in a large bowl.
3. Add lemon juice, olive oil, pepper, and salt in a separate bowl. Whisk.
4. Toss the dressing with the gnocchi mixture and enjoy!

Nutritional information: 350 calories, 35 g carbohydrates, 15 g protein, 15 g fat, and 5 g fiber per serving.

Chipotle Chicken Quinoa Burrito Bowl
(Killeen, 2023a)

Smoky and spicy flavor!

Ingredients

- 1 pound chicken breasts, skinless, boneless, seasoned with chipotle powder
- 1 cup quinoa, cooked
- 1 red bell pepper, diced
- 1/2 onion, diced
- 1 avocado, sliced
- 1/2 cup salsa
- 1/4 cup cilantro, chopped
- lime wedges

Instructions

1. Grill the chicken until it's well cooked.
2. Sauté the bell pepper and onion.
3. Assemble bowls with quinoa, chicken, veggies, avocado, salsa, cilantro, and lime wedges.

Nutritional information: 450 calories, 35 g carbohydrates, 40 g protein, 20 g fat, and 5 g fiber.

White Bean and Avocado Toast
(Seaver, 2023)

Creamy and green niceness in one plate!

Ingredients

- 2 slices whole-wheat bread, toasted
- 1/4 teaspoon garlic powder
- 1/4 avocado, sliced
- salt and pepper to taste
- 1/2 cup white beans, mashed
- 1 tablespoon lemon juice
- tomatoes, red onion, sprouts (as optional toppings)

Instructions

1. Add white beans along with garlic powder, lemon juice, pepper, and salt. Mash these ingredients together.
2. Spread the bean mixture on toast. Top with avocado slices and desired toppings.

Nutritional information: 300 calories, 30 g carbohydrates, 15 g protein, 15 g fat, 8 g fiber.

Roasted Vegetable and Black Bean Tacos
(Fountaine, 2020)

Enjoy fresh garden goodness!

Ingredients

- 1 each of bell pepper, zucchini, onion, all sliced
- 1/2 cup canned black beans, drained and rinsed

- 1 tablespoon olive oil
- 1 teaspoon cumin
- 1/2 teaspoon chili powder
- salt and pepper to taste
- 4 small whole-wheat tortillas
- salsa, avocado, cilantro (optional toppings as desired)

Instructions

1. Toss veggies with olive oil, spices, salt, and pepper. Roast until tender.
2. Warm tortillas.
3. Fill tortillas with roasted veggies, black beans, and desired toppings.

Nutritional information: 350 calories, 40 g carbohydrates, 15 g protein, 10 g fat, and 8 g fiber per serving.

Tomato and Avocado Cheese Sandwich
(Webster, 2023)

Classic comfort brought to your plate!

Ingredients

- 1/2 avocado, sliced
- 1 handful baby spinach
- 2 slices whole-wheat bread, toasted
- 1 tomato, sliced
- 1 low-fat cheese, sliced
- salt and pepper to taste

Instructions

1. Toast bread. Layer avocado, tomato, cheese, and spinach on one slice of bread. Add salt and pepper to taste. Top with a second bread slice.

Nutritional information: 400 calories, 25 g carbohydrates, 15 g protein, 15 g fat, and 5 g fiber.

Weight-Loss Cabbage Soup
(Casner, 2024)

Light and savory delicacy!

Ingredients

- 4 cups vegetable broth
- 1 onion, chopped
- 4 cups cabbage, chopped
- 1 can tomatoes, undrained, diced
- 1 bay leaf
- 1 tablespoon olive oil
- 2 cloves garlic, minced
- salt and pepper to taste

Instructions

1. Heat the oil in a pot over medium heat. Sauté the onion until softened. Add garlic and cook for another minute.
2. Stir in the cabbage, broth, tomatoes, and bay leaf. Add pepper and salt for seasoning. Simmer for 20 minutes.

Nutritional information: 100 calories, 15 g carbohydrates, 5 g protein, 5 g fat, and 5 g fiber per serving.

Ancho Chicken Breast with Black Beans, Bell Peppers, and Scallions (Ansel, 2020)

Pop your taste buds with flavor!

Ingredients

- 1 pound chicken breast, boneless, skinless, and seasoned with ancho chili powder
- 1/2 cup canned black beans, drained and rinsed
- 2 scallions, sliced
- 1 red bell pepper, diced
- 1/2 teaspoon cumin
- 1/2 onion, diced
- salt and pepper to taste
- 1 tablespoon olive oil
- 1/4 teaspoon chili powder

Instructions

1. Grill or bake chicken until cooked through.
2. Add oil to a pan and heat over medium heat. Sauté the bell pepper and onions until they appear softened. Add chili powder, black beans, pepper, cumin, and salt to the pan and stir.
3. Serve the chicken topped with a bean mixture and scallions.

Nutritional information: 400 calories, 30 g carbohydrates, 40 g protein, 15 g fat, and 8 g fiber per serving.

Chocolate Banana Oatmeal
(Eating Well Test Kitchen, 2023)

Sweet and satisfying treat!

Ingredients

- 1/2 cup oats, rolled
- 1 cup dairy or non-dairy milk
- 1/2 banana, sliced
- 1 tablespoon cocoa powder, unsweetened
- 1/4 teaspoon cinnamon, ground
- pinch of salt
- nuts, chia seeds, berries (optional toppings, chopped)

Instructions

1. Combine oats, milk, banana, cocoa powder, cinnamon, and salt in a saucepan. Bring the ingredients to a boil. Lower the heat and simmer for about five minutes. Stir occasionally.
2. Remove from heat and top with desired toppings.

Nutritional information: 300 calories, 40 g carbohydrates, 10 g protein, 10 g fat, 5 g fiber.

Heart-Healthy Recipes That Boost Brain Function

Nourish your body and mind with the following delicious recipes: Packed with brain-boosting ingredients like omega-3s, antioxidants, and healthy fats, these meals are designed to enhance your cognitive function, focus, and overall well-being. Get ready to fuel your brainpower and tantalize your taste buds!

One-Pan Salmon with Roast Asparagus
(Desmazery, n.d.)

Simple and succulent dish!

Ingredients

- 1 pound salmon fillets, skin-on
- 1 bunch asparagus, trimmed
- 1 tablespoon olive oil
- 1/2 teaspoon garlic powder
- 1/4 teaspoon each salt, black pepper

Instructions

1. Preheat the oven to 400 °F (200 °C). Arrange the salmon fillets, skin-side down, on a baking sheet. Toss asparagus with olive oil, garlic powder, salt, and pepper. Add to the baking sheet around the salmon.
2. Roast for 15-20 minutes, or until the salmon is cooked through and flakes easily.

Nutritional information: 450 calories, 15 g carbohydrates, 40 g protein, 25 g fat, and 2 g fiber per serving.

Salmon and Spinach with Tartare Cream
(Good Food Team, n.d.-c)

A creamy and classy blend of ingredients!

Ingredients

- 1 pound salmon fillets
- 1 bag baby spinach

- 1/4 cup Greek yogurt, plain
- 1 tablespoon capers, chopped
- 1 teaspoon Dijon mustard
- 1/4 teaspoon lemon juice
- salt and pepper to taste

Instructions

1. Grill or bake your salmon.
2. Meanwhile, place a pan on medium heat. Wilt spinach.
3. Add Dijon mustard Greek yogurt, capers, pepper, lemon juice, and salt in a bowl. Combine.
4. Serve salmon over spinach with tartare cream on the side.

Nutritional Information: 350 calories, 10 g carbohydrates, 45 g protein, 20 g fat, and 2 g fiber.

Basque-Style Salmon Stew
(Good Food Team, n.d.-a)

Hearty and flavorful dish!

Ingredients

- 1 tablespoon olive oil
- 1 onion, diced
- 2 cloves garlic, minced
- 1 red bell pepper, diced
- 1 can tomatoes, undrained, diced
- 1 cup fish broth
- 1 bay leaf
- 1 pound salmon fillets, cut into chunks
- 1/2 cup peas

- salt and pepper to taste

Instructions

1. Heat the oil in a pot over medium heat. Sauté onion, garlic, and bell pepper until softened.
2. Stir in the tomatoes, broth, and bay leaf, then simmer.
3. Add salmon chunks and peas. Simmer for 10 minutes, or until the salmon is cooked through. Discard the bay leaf.
4. Season with salt and pepper.

Nutritional information: 400 calories, 30 g carbohydrates, 40 g protein, 15 g fat, and 5 g fiber.

Salsa Spaghetti with Sardines
(Buenfeld, n.d.)

Spicy and savory combinations that will jolt your tastebuds!

Ingredients

- 1 cup spaghetti
- 1 can sardines, drained
- 1/2 cup salsa
- 1/4 cup red onion, chopped
- 1/4 cilantro, chopped
- lime wedges

Instructions

1. Drain and flake sardines.
2. Toss cooked spaghetti with salsa, sardines, red onion, and cilantro.

3. Serve with lime wedges.

Nutritional information: 400 calories, 40 g carbohydrates, 25 g protein, 20 g fat, 5 g fiber.

Spiced Lamb Kebabs with Pea and Herb Couscous
(Boggiano, n.d.)

Take an aromatic adventure into new horizons!

Ingredients

- 1 pound lamb, ground
- 1/2 red onion, chopped
- 1 clove garlic, minced
- 1 teaspoon cumin' ground
- 1/2 teaspoon paprika, smoked
- 1/4 teaspoon coriander, ground
- salt and pepper to taste
- 1 cup couscous
- 1 cup peas, frozen
- 1/4 cup fresh parsley, chopped
- 1/4 cup fresh mint, chopped
- 2 tablespoons olive oil
- 1 lemon, juiced

Instructions

1. In a bowl, combine onion, salt, garlic, spices, lamb, and pepper. Mix well and form into small kebabs.
2. Grill or pan-fry kebabs until cooked through.

3. Meanwhile, cook couscous according to package directions. Stir in peas, parsley, mint, olive oil, and lemon juice.
4. Serve kebabs over couscous mixture.

Nutritional information: 450 calories, 35 g carbohydrates, 35 g protein, 20 g fat, and 5 g fiber.

Spicy Yogurt Chicken
(Good Food Team, n.d.-d)

Get a gentle, creamy kick to your gut!

Ingredients

- 1 pound chicken breasts, skinless, cubed
- 1 cup Greek yogurt, plain
- 1 tablespoon curry powder
- salt and pepper to taste
- 1 teaspoon garam masala
- 1/2 teaspoon ginger powder
- 1/4 teaspoon cayenne pepper (adjust as desired)
- 1 onion, diced
- 2 cloves garlic, minced
- 1 tablespoon olive oil
- 1 can tomatoes, undrained, diced
- 1/2 cup chopped cilantro, fresh

Instructions

1. Combine salt, spices, yogurt, and pepper in a bowl and mix well. Marinate your chicken for more than 15 minutes.
2. Heat oil in a pan over medium heat. Sauté the garlic and onion until they are softened.
3. Add the chicken and cook until browned on all sides.
4. Stir in the tomatoes and simmer for 10 minutes.
5. Garnish with cilantro before serving.

Nutritional information: 350 calories, 20 g carbohydrates, 40 g protein, 15 g fat, 3 g fiber.

Chickpea Stew with Tomatoes and Spinach
(Gulati, n.d.)

Delicious one-pot wonder!

Ingredients

- 1 tablespoon olive oil
- 1 onion, diced
- 2 cloves garlic, minced
- 1 can tomatoes, undrained, diced
- 1 can chickpeas, drained and rinsed
- 4 cups vegetable broth
- 1 cup baby spinach
- 1/2 teaspoon cumin
- 1/4 teaspoon smoked paprika
- salt and pepper to taste

Instructions

1. Heat the oil in a pot over medium heat. Sauté the onion and garlic until softened.
2. Add tomatoes, cumin, chickpeas, salt, broth, pepper, and paprika to the pot and bring these ingredients to a boil. Reduce the heat and let the ingredients simmer for 15 minutes.
3. Add spinach and cook until it wilts.

Nutritional information: 300 calories, 40 g carbohydrates, 15 g protein, 5 g fat, 10 g fiber per serving.

Pear and Blueberry Breakfast Bowl
(Good Food Team, n.d.-b)

Get a sweet start to your day!

Ingredients

- 1/2 pear, diced
- 1/2 cup each frozen blueberries
- 1/2 cup cooked rolled oats
- 1/2 unsweetened almond milk
- 1/2 plain Greek yogurt
- 1 tablespoon chia seeds
- 1/4 teaspoon cinnamon, ground
- honey or maple syrup (optional, to taste)

Instructions

1. Layer pear, blueberries, oats, almond milk, yogurt, chia seeds, and cinnamon in a bowl.
2. Drizzle with honey or maple syrup (optional).

Nutritional information: 300 calories, 40 g carbohydrates, 10 g protein, 10 g fat, and 5 g fiber per serving.

Sweet and Healthy Treats

Indulge guilt-free with these delightful treats! I've curated a selection of desserts that satisfy your sweet tooth while adhering to intermittent fasting principles. Packed with heart-healthy ingredients and lower in sugar, these recipes prove that healthy eating can be truly delicious.

Crispy Smashed Apples with Cinnamon Sugar

Enjoy this warm and comforting sweet treat!

Ingredients

- 2 apples, thinly sliced
- 1 tablespoon butter
- 1/4 cup brown sugar
- 1 teaspoon cinnamon, ground

Recipe instructions

1. Preheat the oven to 400°F. Toss apples with butter.
2. Spread apples on a baking sheet and sprinkle with cinnamon sugar.

3. Bake for 20 to 25 minutes, or until tender and crispy.

Nutritional information: 200 calories, 25 g carbohydrates, 1 g protein, 10 g fat, and 2 g fiber. Serve

Pear Cobbler

Rustic and delicious treat!

Ingredients

- 3 pears, thinly sliced
- 1/2 all-purpose flour
- 1/4 cup each rolled oats, brown sugar, cubed cold butter
- 1/4 teaspoon ground cinnamon
- pinch of salt

Instructions

1. Preheat the oven to 375 °F. Arrange the pears in a baking dish.
2. Combine flour, oats, brown sugar, butter, cinnamon, and salt in a bowl until crumbly.
3. Sprinkle crumble over pears and bake for 30–35 minutes, or until golden brown and bubbly.

Nutritional information: 300 calories, 35 g carbohydrates, 2 g protein, 15 g fat.

Individual Strawberry Shortcakes

A miniature fruity delight!

Ingredients

- 1 cup all-purpose flour
- 1 tablespoon sugar
- 1 teaspoon baking powder
- 1/4 teaspoon salt
- 1/4 cup each cubed cold butter, milk, whipped cream
- 1 cup fresh, sliced strawberries

Recipe instructions

1. Preheat your oven to 400 °F. Use a bowl to combine flour, baking powder, sugar, and salt. Add butter until the mixture appears crumbly.
2. Stir in the milk until just combined. Form the dough into 4 small biscuits and place them on a baking sheet.
3. Bake until golden brown for just over 10 minutes. Split biscuits and top with whipped cream and strawberries (optional).

Nutritional information: 350 calories, 40 g carbohydrates, 4 g protein, 15 g fat, 2 g fiber.

Peanut Butter and Jelly Dessert Bars

An easy-to-make treat!

Ingredients

- 1 cup rolled oats
- 1/2 cup each peanut butter, jelly
- 1/4 cup each honey, nuts, chopped

Instructions

1. Line an 8x8-inch baking dish with parchment paper.
2. Combine oats, peanut butter, and honey in a bowl until well-mixed. Press the mixture into the bottom of the baking dish.
3. Spread jelly over the peanut butter layer. Refrigerate for about 30 minutes, then cut into bars.

Nutritional information: 250 calories, 30 g carbohydrates, 5 g protein, 10 g fat, and 2 g fiber per serving.

The Easiest Low-Carb Chocolate Banana Bread Recipe

Indulge guilt-free in this treat!

Ingredients

- 2 ripe bananas, mashed
- 1/2 cup almond flour
- 1/4 cup cocoa powder, unsweetened
- 1 teaspoon baking soda
- 1/4 teaspoon salt
- 2 eggs, beaten

- 1/4 cup each of sugar-free maple syrup, dark chocolate chips

Instructions

1. Warm the oven to 350 °F. Grease a loaf pan.
2. Combine the dry ingredients (flour, cocoa powder, baking soda, and salt) in a bowl.
3. In another bowl, whisk together the mashed bananas, eggs, and maple syrup.
4. Add the wet ingredients to the dry ingredients and mix until just combined. Fold in chocolate chips (optional).
5. Pour the batter into the prepared pan and bake for 40 to 45 minutes.

Nutritional information: 200 calories, 5 g carbohydrates, 5 g protein, 10 g fat per serving.

Healthy Apple Crumble with Pear Recipe

Excite your taste buds with this light & fruity treat!

Ingredients

- 3 apples, sliced
- 1 pear, sliced
- 1/4 cup each rolled oats, chopped walnuts, almond flour, coconut sugar
- 1/4 teaspoon cinnamon
- pinch of salt

Instructions

1. Preheat the oven to 375 °F. Arrange apples and pears in a baking dish.
2. Combine oats, walnuts, flour, sugar, cinnamon, and salt in a bowl. Mix with a fork until crumbly.
3. Sprinkle crumble over the fruit and bake for 25 to 30 minutes, or until golden brown and bubbly.

Nutritional information: 250 calories, 15 g carbohydrates, 3 g protein, 10 g fat, and 5 g fiber per serving.

Peanut Butter Banana Smoothie

Creamy and energizing delicacy!

Ingredients

- 1 banana, frozen
- 1/2 cup dairy or non-dairy milk
- 2 tablespoons peanut butter
- 1 tablespoon Greek yogurt
- 1 teaspoon honey
- 1/4 cup spinach
- ice cubes (as desired)

Instructions

1. Blend all ingredients in a blender until smooth and creamy. Add more milk or ice for the desired consistency.

Nutritional information: 300 calories, 30 g carbohydrates, 15 g protein, 15 g fat, and 5 g fiber per serving.

High-Protein Muffin with Chocolate Chip Banana Nut

Enjoy a delicious, power-packed breakfast!

Ingredients

- 1/2 cup rolled oats
- 1/4 cup each of oat flour, protein powder (chocolate), mashed banana, dairy, or non-dairy milk
- 1 egg, beaten
- 1 tablespoon chia seeds
- 1/4 teaspoon each baking powder, cinnamon
- pinch of salt
- handful each of chopped walnuts, dark chocolate chips

Instructions

1. Preheat the oven to 375 °F. Grease muffin tins.
2. Combine dry ingredients (oats, oat flour, protein powder, baking powder, cinnamon, and salt) in a bowl.
3. In another bowl, whisk together the wet ingredients (banana, milk, egg, and chia seeds).
4. Mix the dry and wet ingredients until well mixed. Mix in nuts and chocolate chips.
5. Divide the batter into muffin tins and bake for 20 to 25 minutes.

Nutritional information: 250 calories, 25 g carbohydrates, 20 g protein, 10 g fats, and 5 g fiber per serving.

No Bake Pumpkin Protein Balls

Simple and tasty!

Ingredients

- 1 cup rolled oats
- 1/2 cup cooked pumpkin puree
- 1/4 cup each protein powder (vanilla or pumpkin spice), almond butter, maple syrup
- 1/4 teaspoon ground cinnamon
- pinch of salt
- chopped nuts, seeds, dark chocolate chips (toppings as desired)

Instructions

1. Use a bowl to mix all ingredients except the toppings. Mix well until a dough forms.
2. Roll dough into balls using slightly damp hands.
3. Refrigerate for about 30 minutes so that the dough becomes firmer.
4. Roll balls in desired toppings, if using.

Nutritional information: 200 calories, 20 g carbohydrates, 15 g proteins, 10 g fat, and 5 g fiber per serving.

Gluten-Free Chocolate Avocado Brownies

Rich and decadent meal!

Ingredients

- 1 ripe avocado, mashed
- 1/2 cup almond flour
- 1/4 cup of each unsweetened cocoa powder, maple syrup, melted coconut oil
- 1 egg, beaten
- 1/2 teaspoon baking powder
- pinch of salt
- chopped nuts, dark chocolate chips, and flaked sea salt as toppings (as desired).

Instructions

1. Preheat your oven to a temperature of 350 °F. Line an 8x8-inch baking dish with parchment paper.
2. In a large bowl, combine mashed avocado, almond flour, cocoa powder, maple syrup, coconut oil, egg, baking powder, and salt. Mix well until smooth.
3. Pour the batter into the prepared baking dish and bake for 20 to 25 minutes.
4. Let cool completely before cutting into squares and topping with the desired ingredients.

Nutritional information: 250 calories, 5 g carbohydrates, 5 g protein, and 20 g fat per serving.

INGREDIENTS AND BENEFITS

Let's explore some healthy ingredients, which are the powerhouses of nutrition that fuel your body and optimize your fasting journey. I reveal the health benefits of each ingredient so that you find it easier to make informed choices when preparing your meals:

Leafy Greens

Leafy greens aren't just salad fillers. They are superfoods that are packed with vitamin K, which is essential for strong bones and blood clotting. Leafy greens are also low in calories and high in fiber, making them ideal for intermittent fasting while also keeping you feeling full. Additionally, the nitrates found in leafy greens can improve blood flow and heart health, thus positively impacting your overall well-being.

Berries

Bursting with vibrant colors, berries aren't just delicious fruits. These tiny fruits are powerful antioxidants packed with protective abilities against free radicals. This property protects your cells and reduces your risk of chronic diseases. And let's not forget their fiber content, which keeps you feeling fuller for much longer, thereby making them a perfect intermittent fasting snack.

Tomatoes

Tomatoes are valuable sources of lycopene, an antioxidant that is linked to a reduced risk of developing certain cancers and heart disease. Their low-calorie, high-fiber content also makes them a fantastic addition to any intermittent fasting meal.

Fatty Fish

Fatty fish varieties, like salmon, tuna, and mackerel, are rich in omega-3 fatty acids. These essential fats are like superheroes for your heart, reducing inflammation and lowering the risk of heart disease. These fish varieties are also packed with high-quality protein.

Whole Grains

Opting for whole wheat bread, brown rice, or quinoa instead of their refined counterparts gives you all the essential nutrients of the entire grain, not just a part of it. This translates to lower cholesterol and blood pressure, thanks to their high fiber content. The fiber content of whole grains also keeps you feeling fuller and more satisfied, making them perfect for intermittent fasting.

Nuts and Seeds

Packed with healthy fats and fiber, these little gems are good for your heart health. They are ideal for intermittent fasting, as they can reduce the risk of heart disease and keep you satisfied for longer.

Avocados

Avocados are more than just tasty toast toppings. They are also rich in monounsaturated fats, which support healthy cholesterol levels. The fiber content of avocados keeps you feeling full and satisfied, making them a great ally for intermittent fasting. Whether you mash them, slice them, or blend them into a smoothie, avocados offer a delicious and nutritious way to boost your health.

TIPS FOR CHOOSING INGREDIENTS

When it comes to nourishing your body, the ingredients you choose make all the difference. For maximum flavor and health benefits, prioritize fresh, seasonal produce. Let your senses guide you. Vibrant colors, fresh aromas, and crisp textures indicate top-notch quality. Opt for whole foods over processed options whenever possible, as they retain their natural nutrients and fiber. Deciphering food labels is also key to choosing the best ingredients. Be mindful of added sugars, sodium, and unhealthy fats. Whenever possible, choose organic options to reduce your exposure to pesticides and chemicals that could negatively affect your health. Also, be sure to embrace seasonal food options, as these are usually at their peak flavor and affordability. Finally, prioritize lean proteins like fish, poultry, and beans for a complete and balanced diet.

This chapter has presented you with a healthy nutritional guide by offering you over 28 different meals that you can prepare to improve your health during your intermittent fast. From brain-boosting recipes to those that promote weight loss, there are many delicious varieties of dishes that you can choose from. I also gave you the ingredients, recipe instructions, and nutritional value of each of these dishes to help you regulate your intake according to your preference. The health benefits of some of the ingredients were also covered in this chapter, while also emphasizing the need to always go for fresh ingredients and opt for seasonal varieties whenever possible. I will help you arrange these meals throughout your days as I share with you a 28-day meal planner in the next chapter.

YOUR 28-DAY PATH TO SUCCESS

"Fasting gets more manageable over time as your body adapts to fueling itself with body fat rather than food."

— JASON FUNG

You might be thinking, "28 days?" Yes, you got that right, but there is no need to get skeptical. While fasting can be a bit challenging as you start, it becomes progressively easier as you continue practicing it. So, you guessed it right—the greatest break-through is to get started. This chapter will provide you with a detailed 28-day meal planner that incorporates the recipes that we described in Chapter 7. It will focus on the letter **E** of the GRACE framework, which stands for Enrich.

THE 28-DAY MEAL PLANNING MADE SIMPLE

It's time to turn Chapter 7 from theory to practical! Learn how you can incorporate various recipes into sustainable meal plans that support your intermittent fasting goals.

Week 1: Adopt Initiation

What will keep you standing during this week is understanding the basics of intermittent fasting, and the nuggets provided in Chapters 1 and 2 will help you with that. Remember your reasons for engaging in intermittent fasting. Could it be because you want to lose weight, attain a better hormonal balance, enhance mental clarity, or increase your energy levels? Understanding your "why" will keep you motivated to continue fasting even when the going gets tough. It's also important to understand the biology behind intermittent fasting—what will be happening in your body when you are either fasting or eating. Remember, this week could be the most difficult part of your fasting plan. The moment you succeed, your body will have adapted to the eating patterns, so the following weeks might be way easier.

During this week, choose two fasting days of your choice and eat for five! This sounds reasonable, right? To begin with, do the 12-hour fast. This means that you could eat from 9:00 a.m. to 9:00 p.m.

Ideally, this week's breakfast should be packed with vegetables. Include whole grains, lean proteins, and colorful vegetables for your lunch and dinner. The table below provides you with suggestions of meals that you can prepare during the eating window, that is, after your fast.

Fasting Days	Breakfast	Lunch	Dinner
Day 1	Tomato and Avocado Cheese Sandwich	Summer Vegetable Gnocchi Salad	Roasted Vegetable and Black Bean Tacos
Day 2	White Bean and Avocado Toast	Chickpea Stew With Tomatoes and Spinach	Balsamic Chicken and Vegetables

You can also use any of the following recipes to replace the ones on the table, just as you deem fit. Get the full recipes in Chapter 7.

- Chile-Lime Tilapia with Corn Saute
- Seared Salmon with Pistachio Gremolata
- Balsamic Chicken and Vegetables
- Oven-Roasted Salmon with Charred Lemon Vinaigrette
- Chicken Kebabs

Week 2: Explore the Waters and Savor the Adventure

Welcome to Week 2 of your fasting plan. At this point, add just two more hours to your fasting window so that it stretches for 14 hours. Even though we assume that your body is now getting more comfortable with fasting, it's crucial for you to listen to its cues and respond accordingly. Be sure to keep yourself hydrated and include whole foods that are nutritious when you break your fast. The table below presents the provisional meal plan that you can use during your eating window.

Fasting Days	Breakfast	Lunch	Dinner
Day 1	Pear and Blueberry Breakfast Bowl	Weight-Loss Cabbage Soup	Chipotle Chicken Quinoa Burrito Bowl
Day 2	Chocolate Banana Oatmeal	Kale and White Bean Potpie with Chive Biscuits	Salsa Spaghetti With Sardines

Here are more recipes that you can include, in case you want to swap the ones that are on the table. Find the full recipe in Chapter 7.

- Roasted Asparagus, Fish, and Bay Leaves
- Hot Honey-Roasted Salmon and Radishes
- Salmon with Lemon and Herbs
- Skillet Lasagna

Week 3: Master the Art of Fasting and Plant Power

Brace yourself for the 15-hour fast this week! This could mean eating from 9 a.m. to 6 p.m. Always aim to eat more plant food this week. Hydrating remains an important aspect of your fasting routine. Be patient with yourself as you go and gather your resilience. It's been two weeks since you started intermittent fasting; you conquered, and there is nothing that can stop you now! To make it easier for you to select your meals for your eating windows, I compiled the table below.

Fasting Days	Breakfast	Lunch	Dinner
Day 1	Salmon-Stuffed Avocados	Chickpea Stew With Tomatoes and Spinach	Salmon with Lemon and Herbs
Day 2	Pear and Blueberry Breakfast Bowl	Spiced Lamb Kebabs With Pea and Herb Couscous	Roasted Asparagus, Fish, and Bay Leaves

Here are more recipes that can increase the variety of meals that you can choose from. Feel free to replace the ones on the table as you deem fit. All recipes are available in Chapter 7.

- Kale and White Bean Potpie with Chive Biscuits
- Summer Vegetable Gnocchi Salad
- Chipotle Chicken Quinoa Burrito Bowl
- White Bean and Avocado Toast
- Roasted Vegetable and Black Bean Tacos

Week 4: Optimize and Thrive, Seafood, and Spiralize

Congratulations! You have just entered the final week of this intermittent fasting challenge. This time around, you are doing a 16-hour fast. You can consider starting your eating window at 9 a.m. and finishing at 5 p.m. This is a week during which you should optimize your fasting routine. Try different things and determine what works best for you. For instance, you could add some exercises or adjust your fasting windows and meals. In this section, you will find some recipes that you can consider during this final week. The full recipes for the meals are described in Chapter 7.

Fasting Days	Breakfast	Lunch	Dinner
Day 1	Tomato and Avocado Cheese Sandwich	Spicy Yogurt Chicken	Seared Salmon with Pistachio Gremolata
Day 2	Spiced Lamb Kebabs With Pea and Herb Couscous	Chile-Lime Tilapia with Corn Saute	Oven-Roasted Salmon with Charred Lemon Vinaigrette

FASTING FORWARD: ADJUSTING FOR SUCCESS

To increase your chances of being successful in attaining your goals for intermittent fasting, leave room for flexibility. It's important that you pay special attention to how your body responds to fasting as you progress. If, for example, you realize that the hunger cues are interfering with your day-to-day activities, you can reduce the fasting window until your body adjusts. Alternatively, eating heavy meals during the feasting window could increase your energy reserves, thereby helping you to push for longer without eating. In some cases, hydrating yourself as much as possible could be all you need!

There are advantages that come with embracing flexibility when practicing intermittent fasting. Just to mention a few, flexibility

- allows you to adjust the size of your meals as necessary.
- can help boost your metabolism.
- makes intermittent fasting more sustainable, considering that less strictness makes the practice easier.
- gives you the leverage to listen to your body's needs, so you won't neglect them in the process.

Strategies for Making Adjustments

If you had already started your intermittent fasting journey, you might have been wondering how best you could make relevant adjustments. Well, there are plenty of ideas available, and we will explore some of them in this section. Even if you have yet to start intermittent fasting, these nuggets remain handy:

- **Adjust the eating window:** For example, if you feel that starting with the 12-hour fasting window feels so overwhelming for you, you could try the 10-hour window. Similarly, if you feel that you have become so used to the 12-hour window, stepping up to a bigger fasting window could be the way to go.
- **Identify your fasting rhythm:** Your fasting rhythm could mean the length of your fasting and eating windows. It could also refer to the frequency at which you fast, say, in a week. Find out the fasting rhythm that works for you and stick to it. Consistency is power.
- **Modify your portion sizes:** Depending on the intensity of hunger cues, you can increase or reduce the portion sizes of your food. It could be the same oatmeal that you had

planned to eat for breakfast, but you changed the portion size.

- **Swap the recipes:** Sometimes, you need to completely change the recipes. For example, instead of a recipe with chicken breast as the source of your lean proteins, you could go more vegan by replacing it with chickpeas.
- **Keep busy during your fasting periods:** You're more likely to feel hungry when you are idle. Give yourself targets for completing tasks so that you keep your hands and mind busy. Before you know it, the fasting window will be over!
- **Eat nutrient-dense foods during your eating periods:** When it's time to eat, make sure your meal plan is nutrient-packed. This will keep you healthy, even though you're fasting intermittently.
- **Listen to your body:** Take time to pay attention to your body's cues. What is your body saying? Is it comfortable? Are you stretching it too hard? Whatever the case might be, adjust accordingly.

This chapter marks a smooth transition from the theoretical information provided in Chapter 7. It provides you with practical meal plans and options that are not only feasible but sustainable, too. The meal plans that are presented in this chapter take you through the process of upgrading your fasting by progressively increasing the non-eating hours. Always remember to listen to your body so that you can make relevant adjustments to fasting schedules, meal plans, portion sizes, or even daily activities. You see, the chapters in this book are well-knit together to give you the GRACE framework for intermittent fasting. Now, it's time for you to practice what you learned and reap the benefits.

Congratulations on making it to the end of this intermittent fasting guide!

CONCLUSION

Age gracefully with intermittent fasting! Increase your energy levels and effectively manage your weight gain through intermittent fasting. Not only that, but this practice also reduces inflammation while improving your hormonal balance, focus, and cognitive function. It's up to you to choose the type of intermittent fasting that works best for you. Here are some of the available options:

- **16:8 method:** In this case, you fast for 16 hours and eat for 8 hours a day.
- **12-hour overnight fasting:** Here, the bulk of the fasting is done while you're sleeping.
- **14:10 method:** This involves a 14-hour fasting window and a 10-hour eating one.
- **Eat-stop-eat method:** You select two days of the week, during which you will fast for the whole 24 hours.
- **5:2 method:** In this case, you fast two days of the week. On the fasting days, you don't necessarily have to refrain from eating for 24 hours.

Any of these methods will see you reaping the health-related benefits of intermittent fasting. This is not a fairy tale, there are people who will not hesitate to bet their 20 cents on intermittent fasting —Debbie Rose is one of them. With a weight of 298 pounds, the then-71-year-old Debbie was faced with the risk of having to use a wheelchair for the rest of her life. The only viable option at her disposal was losing weight, but how would she do that? She felt so overwhelmed and hopeless. Debbie came across the answer to her worry as she was watching a show about intermittent fasting on television. Debbie felt that this was her *"eureka"* moment, and she was ready to try intermittent fasting as a weight-loss strategy. To get started, Debbie decided to miss at least one meal a day, and breakfast was her best pick. Over time, Debbie's weight dropped to 181 pounds—a whopping 117 pounds were gone! Intermittent fasting saved Debbie from having to sit in a wheelchair for the rest of her life. Try this practice and let it save you from hormonal imbalances, cognitive decline, compromised focus, and an increased risk of conditions like diabetes and heart disease.

As you turn the last pages of this book, remember that it's just the beginning of your journey with intermittent fasting. You now hold the keys to a transformative approach to health—one that respects your body's wisdom and the changes it goes through after 50. Don't wait another day! Embrace the guidance, tap into the energy, and balance your hormones. Let this book be the catalyst for a healthier, happier you. Take the first step into a world where age is just a number and vitality is your daily experience. Begin your intermittent fasting journey today, and let your next years be your best years!

Keeping the Game Alive: Sharing is Caring

"Helping one person might not change the whole world, but it could change the world for one person."

— *UNKNOWN*

You Did It!

Congratulations on completing the book and gaining valuable insights into maintaining health as a woman over 50. Now, you can help others start their journey.

Your Review Matters:

Share your experiences and inspire someone else to begin their path to better health. Your review could:

- Encourage another to try intermittent fasting.
- Offer the courage to make healthy changes.
- Help find clarity and balance.
- Motivate overcoming challenges.
- Inspire happier, healthier lives.

Leave a Review in Seconds.

Your words can light the way for others. Thank you for contributing to our community and becoming a beacon of hope and guidance.

REFERENCES

Ackerman, C. E. (2019, June 26). *58 science-based mindful eating exercises and tips.* PositivePsychology.com. https://positivepsychology.com/mindful-eating-exercises/

Al Qudsi, F. (2022, December 8). *Intermittent Fasting for Women Over 50: Key things to know.* FuadFit. https://www.fuadfit.com/blog/intermittent-fasting-for-women-over-50-key-things-to-know

Ansel, K. (2020, March 5). *Ancho chicken breast with black beans, bell peppers, and scallions.* EatingWell. https://www.eatingwell.com/recipe/256508/ancho-chicken-breast-with-black-beans-bell-peppers-scallions/

Berg, E. (2018, January 22). *5 Reasons Why You Feel Tired On Keto Diet! – Dr. Berg on intermittent fasting and fatigue.* www.youtube.com. https://www.youtube.com/watch?v=yvO4GC2fA_M

Berg, E. (2023, August 31). *Dealing with intermittent fasting fatigue: 5 common causes.* www.drberg.com. https://www.drberg.com/blog/the-5-reasons-you-get-tired-on-intermittent-fasting

BHG Kitchen. (2016, August 18). *Skillet lasagna.* Better Homes & Gardens. https://www.bhg.com/recipe/skillet-lasagna/

BHG Test Kitchen. (2011, June 14). *Balsamic chicken and vegetables.* Better Homes & Gardens. https://www.bhg.com/recipe/chicken/balsamic-chicken-and-vegetables/

BHG Test Kitchen. (2017). *Seared salmon with pistachio gremolata.* Better Homes & Gardens. https://www.bhg.com/recipe/seared-salmon-with-pistachio-gremolata/

BHG Test Kitchen. (2017, April 19). *Roasted asparagus, fish, and bay leaves.* Better Homes & Gardens. https://www.bhg.com/recipe/roasted-asparagus-fish-and-bay-leaves/

BHG Test Kitchen. (2018). *Chile-lime tilapia with corn sauté.* Better Homes and Gardens. https://www.bhg.com/recipe/chile-lime-tilapia-with-corn-saut/

Bjarnadottir, A. (2019, June 19). *Mindful eating 101: A beginner's guide.* Healthline Media. https://www.healthline.com/nutrition/mindful-eating-guide

Boggiano, A. (n.d.). *Spiced lamb kebabs with pea & herb couscous.* Good Food. Retrieved March 28, 2024, from https://www.bbcgoodfood.com/recipes/spiced-lamb-kebabs-pea-herb-couscous

Buenfeld, S. (n.d.). *Salsa spaghetti with sardines*. Good Food. Retrieved March 28, 2024, from https://www.bbcgoodfood.com/recipes/salsa-spaghetti-sardines

Cafiero, K. (2020, February 3). *A Day in the Life of an Intermittent Faster*. RVNAhealth for Lifelong Care and Wellness - for Lifelong Care and Wellness. https://rvna health.org/news/a-day-in-the-life-of-an-intermittent-faster/

Capritto, A. (2024). *How to start exercising when you're 50 and older*. CNET. https://www.cnet.com/health/fitness/how-to-start-exercising-in-your-50s-and-beyond/

Casner, C. (2023, September 19). *Crispy smashed apples with cinnamon sugar*. EatingWell. https://www.eatingwell.com/recipe/7922087/crispy-smashed-apples-with-cinnamon-sugar/

Casner, C. (2024, February 27). *Weight-loss cabbage soup*. EatingWell. https://www.eatingwell.com/recipe/269488/cabbage-diet-soup/

Cienfuegos, S., Corapi, S., Gabel, K., Ezpeleta, M., Kalam, F., Lin, S., Pavlou, V., & Varady, K. A. (2022). Effect of intermittent fasting on reproductive hormone levels in females and males: A review of human trials. *Nutrients, 14*(11), 2343. https://doi.org/10.3390/nu14112343

Coppa, C. (2020, February 27). *10 mistakes you can make while intermittent fasting*. EatingWell. https://www.eatingwell.com/article/7676144/mistakes-you-can-make-while-intermittent-fasting/

DeCesaris, L. (2023, January 18). *How intermittent fasting affects women's hormones*. Rupa Health. https://www.rupahealth.com/post/how-intermittent-fasting-affects-womens-hormones

Desmazery, B. (n.d.). *One-pan salmon with roast asparagus*. BBC Good Food. https://www.bbcgoodfood.com/recipes/one-pan-salmon-roast-asparagus

Dodd, K. (2021, January 15). *High protein muffin*. High Calorie Recipes. https://highcalorierecipes.com/high-protein-muffin/

DoFasting Editorial. (2022, March 25). *7 tips on how to curb hunger while fasting*. DoFasting Blog. https://dofasting.com/blog/how-to-curb-hunger-while-fasting/

Donnelly, J. E., Smith, B., Jacobsen, D. J., Kirk, E., DuBose, K., Hyder, M., Bailey, B., & Washburn, R. (2004). The role of exercise for weight loss and maintenance. *Best Practice & Research Clinical Gastroenterology, 18*(6), 1009–1029. https://doi.org/10.1016/j.bpg.2004.06.022

Downing, D. (2022, November 3). *How women's bodies change with age: 30, 40, 50 & beyond*. Canyon Ranch. https://www.canyonranch.com/well-stated/post/a-womans-changing-body/

Eating Well Test Kitchen. (2023, September 20). *Chocolate banana oatmeal*. EatingWell. https://www.eatingwell.com/recipe/251103/chocolate-banana-oatmeal/

Egypt Today Staff. (2023, April 3). *5 tips to improve your concentration and productivity while fasting.* EgyptToday. https://www.egypttoday.com/Article/6/123519/5-Tips-to-Improve-Your-Concentration-and-Productivity-While-Fasting

Fasting for mental clarity: Enhance your brain function. (2023, April 24). Santosh Yoga Institute. https://santoshyogainstitute.com/fasting-for-mental-clarity/

Fiacco, S., Mernone, L., & Ehlert, U. (2020). Psychobiological indicators of the subjectively experienced health status - findings from the Women 40+ Healthy Aging Study. *BMC Women's Health, 20*(1). https://doi.org/10.1186/s12905-020-0888-x

findthegood123. (2023, October 17). *Looking to hear from older women (49+) who did IF. Would love to hear both successes and failures.* Reddit.com. https://www.reddit.com/r/intermittentfasting/comments/179w89s/looking_to_hear_from_older_women_49_who_did_if/?rdt=60258

Fountaine, S. (2020, June 23). *Roasted vegetable and black bean tacos.* EatingWell. https://www.eatingwell.com/recipe/257722/roasted-vegetable-black-bean-tacos/

Freytag, C. (2022, September 22). *Must-do strength training moves for women over 50.* Verywell Fit. https://www.verywellfit.com/must-do-strength-training-women-over-50-3498202

Garone, S. (2023, July 10). *Intermittent Fasting versus Calorie Counting: Which is more effective for weight loss?* Health. https://www.health.com/intermittent-fasting-vs-calorie-counting-weight-loss-7557026

Gateway Region YMCA. (2019, June 14). *Best exercises for women over 50.* Gwrymca.org. https://gwrymca.org/blog/best-exercises-women-over-50

Gellman, A. (2023, September 19). *Salmon-stuffed avocados.* EatingWell. https://www.eatingwell.com/recipe/270549/salmon-stuffed-avocados/

Good Food Is Good Medicine. (2022, February 4). *Intermittent fasting: Benefits, how it works, and is it right for you?* Good-Food. https://health.ucdavis.edu/blog/good-food/intermittent-fasting-benefits-how-it-works-and-is-it-right-for-you/2022/02

Good Food Team. (n.d.-a). *Basque-style salmon stew.* BBC Good Food. https://www.bbcgoodfood.com/recipes/basque-style-salmon-stew

Good Food Team. (n.d.-b). *Pear and blueberry breakfast bowl.* BBC Good Food. https://www.bbcgoodfood.com/recipes/pear-blueberry-breakfast-bowl

Good Food Team. (n.d.-c). *Salmon and spinach with tartare cream.* Good Food. Retrieved March 28, 2024, from https://www.bbcgoodfood.com/recipes/salmon-spinach-tartare-cream

Good Food Team. (n.d.-d). *Spicy yogurt chicken.* BBC Good Food. https://www.bbcgoodfood.com/recipes/spicy-yogurt-chicken

Gorin, A. (2022, June 17). *Gluten-free chocolate avocado brownies.* Plant Based with

Amy. https://plantbasedwithamy.com/avocado-chocolate-brownies-with-prunes

Gracia, Z. (2022, March 30). *10 intermittent fasting mistakes people make and how to avoid them.* BetterMe Blog. https://betterme.world/articles/intermittent-fasting-mistakes/

Grubb, J. (2024). *Fitness and nutrition for men over 35. Jason Grubb Fitness.* www.jasongrubb.com. https://www.jasongrubb.com/blog/

Guerra, L. (2024). *Simple ways to avoid hunger while fasting: 10 steps.* WikiHow. https://www.wikihow.com/Avoid-Hunger-While-Fasting

Gulati, R. (n.d.). *Chickpea stew with tomatoes & spinach.* BBC Good Food. https://www.bbcgoodfood.com/recipes/chickpeas-tomatoes-spinach

Gunnars, K. (2017, June 4). *What is intermittent fasting? Explained in simple terms.* Healthline. https://www.healthline.com/nutrition/what-is-intermittent-fasting#about-intermittent-fasting

Gunnars, K. (2019, July 22). *11 myths about fasting and meal frequency.* Healthline Media. https://www.healthline.com/nutrition/11-myths-fasting-and-meal-frequency

Gunnars, K. (2020, April 20). *Intermittent fasting 101: The ultimate beginner's guide.* Healthline. https://www.healthline.com/nutrition/intermittent-fasting-guide

Gunnars, K. (2020a, January 1). *6 popular ways to do intermittent fasting.* Healthline. https://www.healthline.com/nutrition/6-ways-to-do-intermittent-fasting

Gunnars, K. (2021, May 13). *10 evidence-based health benefits of intermittent fasting.* Healthline. https://www.healthline.com/nutrition/10-health-benefits-of-intermittent-fasting

Harlan, C. (2016, July 6). *8 women who successfully lost weight after menopause.* Prevention. https://www.prevention.com/weight-loss/g20434709/success-stories-weight-loss-after-menopause/

Hastings, K. (2023, October 3). *Intermittent fasting myths.* LifeMD. https://lifemd.com/learn/intermittent-fasting-myths

Hu, Y., Ji, G., Li, G., Manza, P., Zhang, W., Wang, J., Lv, G., He, Y., Zhang, Z., Yuan, K., von Deneen, K. M., Chen, A., Cui, G., Wang, H., Wiers, C. E., Volkow, N. D., Nie, Y., Zhang, Y., & Wang, G.-J. (2020). Brain connectivity, and hormonal and behavioral correlates of sustained weight loss in obese patients after laparoscopic sleeve gastrectomy. *Cerebral Cortex, 31*(2), 1284–1295. https://doi.org/10.1093/cercor/bhaa294

Hurwitz, K., & Berry, E. (2022, May 8). *Heart-healthy recipes that can be on the table in under 30 minutes.* Woman's Day. https://www.womansday.com/food-recipes/food-drinks/g2176/hearty-healthy-recipes/?slide=6

Johns Hopkins Medicine. (2021a). *Intermittent fasting: What is it, and how does it work?*

Johns Hopkins Medicine. https://www.hopkinsmedicine.org/health/wellness-and-prevention/intermittent-fasting-what-is-it-and-how-does-it-work

Kang, J., Shi, X., Fu, J., Li, H., Ma, E., & Chen, W. (2022). Effects of an intermittent fasting 5:2 plus program on body weight in Chinese adults with overweight or obesity: A pilot study. *Nutrients, 14*(22), 4734. https://doi.org/10.3390/nu14224734

Kanukuntla, J. (2024, January 4). *Intermittent Fasting Do's and Don'ts: Common mistakes to avoid.* Continentalhospitals.com. https://continentalhospitals.com/blog/intermittent-fasting-dos-and-donts-common-mistakes-to-avoid/

Keenan, S., Cooke, M. B., Chen, W. S., Wu, S., & Belski, R. (2022). The Effects of Intermittent Fasting and Continuous Energy Restriction with Exercise on Cardiometabolic Biomarkers, Dietary Compliance, and Perceived Hunger and Mood: Secondary outcomes of a randomised, controlled trial. *Nutrients, 14*(15), 3071. https://doi.org/10.3390/nu14153071

Kerr, M. (2022, January 19). *Exercise and weight loss: Importance, benefits and examples.* Healthline. https://www.healthline.com/health/exercise-and-weight-loss

Killeen, B. L. (2023a, September 19). *Chipotle chicken quinoa burrito bowl.* EatingWell. https://www.eatingwell.com/recipe/254609/chipotle-chicken-quinoa-burrito-bowl/

Killeen, B. L. (2023b, September 19). *Kale and white bean potpie with chive biscuits.* EatingWell. https://www.eatingwell.com/recipe/251252/kale-white-bean-potpie-with-chive-biscuits/

Kim, J. (2023, September 23). *Individual strawberry shortcakes.* EatingWell. https://www.eatingwell.com/recipe/7901863/individual-strawberry-shortcakes/

Kristi. (2020, November 26). *Easy apple pear crisp.* Carrots & Cookies. https://carrotsandcookies.com/healthy-apple-crumble-recipe

Kubala, J. (2023, March 31). *Is fasting safe for women over 50?* Mindbodygreen. https://www.mindbodygreen.com/articles/intermittent-fasting-for-women-over-50

Kuta, A. (2024). *The best balance exercises to do as you age.* Hospital for Special Surgery. https://www.hss.edu/article_balance-exercises.asp

Leonard, J. (2020, April 16). *7 ways to do intermittent fasting: Best methods and quick tips.* Medical News Today. https://www.medicalnewstoday.com/articles/322293

Li, C., Xing, C., Zhang, J., Zhao, H., Shi, W., & He, B. (2021). Eight-hour time-restricted feeding improves endocrine and metabolic profiles in women with anovulatory polycystic ovary syndrome. *Journal of Translational Medicine, 19*(19). https://doi.org/10.1186/s12967-021-02817-2

Link, R. (2018, September 4). *16/8 intermittent fasting: A beginner's guide.* Healthline;

Healthline Media. https://www.healthline.com/nutrition/16-8-intermittent-fasting

MD, K. S. (2017, September 24). *Intermittent fasting: How it energizes my true life.* Karyn Shanks MD. https://www.karynshanksmd.com/2017/09/24/intermittent-fasting-how-it-energizes-my-true-life/

Medical, R. (2024). *How do hormones change as i age?* Rejuvime Medical. https://www.rejuvimemedical.com/blog/how-do-hormones-change-as-i-age/

Moye, E. (2019, October 25). *Pumpkin protein balls: No-bake, gluten-free, vegan option.* Hello Spoonful. https://www.hellospoonful.com/no-bake-pumpkin-protein-balls/

Nast, C. (2023a, April 27). *7 ways to be more mindful without meditating.* SELF. https://www.self.com/story/best-mindfulness-exercises

Nast, C. (2023b, July 4). *3 reasons why intermittent fasting is better than cutting calories, according to an expert.* Vogue. https://www.vogue.com/article/intermittent-fasting-better-than-cutting-calories

National Library of Medicine. (n.d.). *MedlinePlus.* Medlineplus.gov. https://medlineplus.gov/

Nazish, N. (2024). *10 intermittent fasting myths you should stop believing.* Forbes. https://www.forbes.com/sites/nomanazish/2021/06/30/10-intermittent-fasting-myths-you-should-stop-believing/?sh=2b0f02e2335b

Nemetz, A. (2023, July 9). *"I'm 71, and intermittent fasting saved me from a wheelchair — plus I lost 121 lbs!"* Woman's World. https://www.womansworld.com/posts/diets/intermittent-fasting-for-seniors

O'Brien, D. (2023, September 19). *Summer vegetable gnocchi salad.* EatingWell. https://www.eatingwell.com/recipe/280001/summer-vegetable-gnocchi-salad/

Orlowski, M. (2022, July 4). *Peanut butter banana smoothie.* High Calorie Recipes. https://highcalorierecipes.com/peanut-butter-banana-smoothie/

Palinski-Wade, E. (2021, May 26). *The easiest low-carb chocolate banana bread recipe.* Erin Palinski-Wade. https://erinpalinski.com/low-carb-keto-chocolate-banana-bread-recipe

Pandey, N. (2023, April 24). *How meditation can help with intermittent fasting.* Www.linkedin.com. https://www.linkedin.com/pulse/how-meditation-can-help-intermittent-fasting-nitesh-pandey/

Perri, L. (2020, October 14). *Salmon with lemon and herbs.* Better Homes & Gardens. https://www.bhg.com/recipe/salmon-with-lemon-and-herbs/

Piedmont Healthcare. (2024). *Why metabolism slows as you age.* Www.piedmont.org. https://www.piedmont.org/living-real-change/why-metabolism-slows-as-you-age

Prendergast, C. (2022, December 7). *Exercise warmup for seniors.* Physio Ed. https://physioed.com/exercise-warmup-for-seniors/

Quora. (2019). *How was your experience treating arthritis with 3-day fasting?* Quora. https://www.quora.com/How-was-your-experience-treating-arthritis-with-3-day-fasting

Ravussin, E., Beyl, R. A., Poggiogalle, E., Hsia, D. S., & Peterson, C. M. (2019). Early time-restricted feeding reduces appetite and increases fat oxidation but does not affect energy expenditure in humans. *Obesity, 27*(8), 1244–1254. https://doi.org/10.1002/oby.22518

RD, N. G. (2023, August 21). *How to pair mindful eating with mindful fasting.* Zero Longevity. https://zerolongevity.com/blog/how-to-pair-mindful-eating-with-mindful-fasting/

Read, W. (2024, February 5). *28 Day Challenge For Weight Loss - Lose weight with 28 day fasting challenge.* Lasta. https://lasta.app/28-day-fasting-challenge-unleash-your-potential-for-a-healthier-happier-you/?fbclid=IwAR29AV3P8wSlgfK7EqPqmw__28syuAntgfRufywc28plJiSwFxluBeSEwG4

Richard, B. (2018). *Changes in the body with aging.* Merck Manuals Consumer Version; Merck Manuals. https://www.merckmanuals.com/home/older-people%E2%80%99s-health-issues/the-aging-body/changes-in-the-body-with-aging

Ruscio, M. (2022, December 2). *Intermittent fasting for women over 50: Your guide for success - Dr. Michael Ruscio, DC.* Drruscio.com. https://drruscio.com/fasting-for-women-over-50/

Seaver, V. (2023, September 19). *White bean and avocado toast.* EatingWell. https://www.eatingwell.com/recipe/261611/white-bean-avocado-toast/

Shah, M. (2022, August 2). *A comparison of intermittent fasting and other diets.* HealthifyMe. https://www.healthifyme.com/blog/intermittent-fasting-and-other-diets/

Shaw, L. (2019, May 31). *The best exercise program for women over 50.* Livestrong. https://www.livestrong.com/article/446426-the-best-exercise-program-for-women-over-50/

Sheff, T. (2018, June 23). *Easy chicken kebabs.* Cooktoria. https://cooktoria.com/easy-chicken-kebabs/

Singhal, G. (2023, September 15). *12 expert tips for mastering intermittent fasting: Transformative wellness voyage.* Www.linkedin.com. https://www.linkedin.com/pulse/12-expert-tips-mastering-intermittent-fasting-wellness-garv-singhal/

Smith, J. (2023, September 19). *Pear cobbler.* EatingWell. https://www.eatingwell.com/recipe/280783/pear-cobbler/

Stanton, B. (2021). *How to choose an intermittent fasting schedule.* Carb Manager. https://www.carbmanager.com/article/yoherxeaaceazayu/how-to-choose-an-intermittent-fasting-schedule

Stevens, G. (2019). *Success stories.* Gin Stephens, Author and Intermittent Faster.

https://www.ginstephens.com/success-stories.html

Susan Anne Metz. (2021, November 23). *Reanimation in retirement: Fae Olson.* Intermittent Fasting Success. https://intermittentfastingsuccess.com/reanimation-in-retirement/

The Silhouette Clinic. (2023, November 7). *Fasting for weight loss over 50: Optimizing weight loss.* The Silhouette Clinic. https://thesilhouetteclinic.com/fasting-for-weight-loss-over-50/

The University of Illinois. (2022, October 25). *New data on how intermittent fasting affects female hormones.* Today.uic.edu. https://today.uic.edu/new-data-on-how-intermittent-fasting-affects-female-hormones/

The University of Illinois. (2023, August 3). *Research shows that intermittent fasting is safe and effective.* Today.uic.edu. https://today.uic.edu/benefits-intermittent-fasting-research/

University of Illinois. (2021, October 11). *Research review shows intermittent fasting works for weight loss, health changes.* Today.uic.edu. https://today.uic.edu/research-review-shows-intermittent-fasting-works-for-weight-loss-health-changes/

Vetter, C. (2024). *Intermittent fasting: What can you eat or drink?* Zoe.com. https://zoe.com/learn/what-to-eat-or-drink-while-intermittent-fasting

Wang, Y., & Wu, R. (2022). The effect of fasting on human metabolism and psychological health. *Disease Markers, 2022*(26), 1–7. https://doi.org/10.1155/2022/5653739

WebMD Editorial Contributors. (2021, September 27). *What to know about intermittent fasting for women after 50.* WebMD. https://www.webmd.com/healthy-aging/what-to-know-about-intermittent-fasting-for-women-after-50

Webster, K. (2023, September 19). *Tomato-and-avocado cheese sandwich.* EatingWell. https://www.eatingwell.com/recipe/260715/tomato-avocado-cheese-sandwich/

WeFast. (n.d.). *The 8 different methods of intermittent fasting - WeFast.* Www.wefast.care. https://www.wefast.care/articles/8-different-methods-intermittent-fasting

Welton, S., Minty, R., O'Driscoll, T., Willms, H., Poirier, D., Madden, S., & Kelly, L. (2020). Intermittent fasting and weight loss. *Canadian Family Physician, 66*(2), 117–125. https://www.ncbi.nlm.nih.gov/pmc/articles/PMC7021351/

Willard, C. (2019, January 17). *6 Ways to practice mindful eating.* Mindful. https://www.mindful.org/6-ways-practice-mindful-eating/

Woman Day's Kitchen. (2019, October 21). *Oven-roasted salmon with charred lemon vinaigrette.* Woman's Day. https://www.womansday.com/food-recipes/food-drinks/a29464781/oven-roasted-salmon-with-charred-lemon-vinaigrette-recipe/

Yautz, L. (2021, March 31). *Peanut butter and jelly dessert bars: Heart healthy!* Being Nutritious. https://beingnutritious.com/peanut-butter-and-jelly-dessert-bars/

Manufactured by Amazon.ca
Acheson, AB

14810681R00096